EXERCISE
As You Grow Older

EXERCISE As You Grow Older

Naomi Lederach
Nona Kauffman
Beth Lederach

Good Books

Intercourse, Pennsylvania 17534

This book is not meant to replace the services of a physician.
Any application of the recommendations set forth in the
following pages is at the reader's discretion and sole risk.

Table of Contents

Introduction

Exercise can mean different things to different groups of people. For young adults it may mean getting in shape, body sculpturing, or possibly even a social event at an exercise club. For people in their middle years, as I am, exercise usually means a way to maintain general fitness and cardiovascular conditioning. For older adults exercise might be viewed as a way to maintain flexibility, remain independent, and for some, decrease the debilitating effects of chronic degenerative disease processes. Unfortunately, for many people exercise has a negative connotation. Those of us who were required to take gym courses or enroll in physical training in school remember exercise as prescribed by these courses as a joyless chore. Many other people view exercise as a strenuous activity requiring skills and commitment beyond their abilities.

One of the important messages of this book is that exercise can and should be fun. Just as important is the fact that exercise can be practiced by anyone, of either sex, and at any age. Of course, health and physical limitations need to be considered, particularly by older people who are just beginning an exercise program. Virtually everyone, however, given the proper medical advice and guidance, can exercise and can use exercise to improve the quality of their lives.

I feel that another important message of this book is the importance of staying active throughout life. This idea is beautifully illustrated by Grandmother Kauffman. I have also had good role models in my own family to illustrate the importance of regular physical activity for older people. A great-grandfather of mine used to routinely walk from Reading to Pottsville, Pennsylvania, even into his late 80s, to visit his family. A very dear aunt, who died at the age of 88, lived independently and gardened right up to her death. I have very vivid memories of her being on the news when, in her late 80s, she and my uncle were picketing the local agency on aging because they felt that the officials were more concerned about maintaining their relatively high salaries than in providing needed services to the elderly people in their community.

Of course, not everyone can live into their 80s and 90s and many people who do live that long are restricted by chronic disease or other disabilities. And, while exercise may be only a minor contributor to good health, regular exercise can help maximize activity levels, prevent the progression of chronic degenerative diseases if done properly, and give a sense of well-being. Most of my patients who exercise don't do so because they think it is good for them; rather they exercise because doing so makes them feel good. The approach to exercise discussed in this book is sound and should be able to be used by the vast majority of older people.

—*Ted Kantner, M.D.*
Milton S. Hershey Medical Center,
Pennsylvania State University College of Medicine,
Hershey, Pennsylvania

1 Three Is Not a Crowd

We are three normal people writing this book, from three generations. We are quite ordinary people, too. And that's who this book is for—ordinary people. We also believe it is ordinary people who can do extraordinary things when they are encouraged and inspired. They may say to themselves, "Well, if they can do it, so can I."

Let us introduce ourselves. Beth is the youngest, in her twenties, daughter of Naomi and granddaughter of Nona. Naomi is in her fifties, daughter of Nona and also a grandmother. Nona (Grandma) is 87, a grandmother and great-grandmother. She is the extraordinary one, who has decided that, although she fully intends to die some day, she will not stop living now. She has given aging a good name.

This book evolved because of our conviction that as ordinary people, age does not always have to mean decline. We have seen this in our family. Admittedly, there are diseases and illnesses that are part of the experience of many people. But we are speaking to people, men and women, regardless of age, who are relatively healthy, who *could*, if they would, be more active and feel better about themselves and be even healthier, too.

Growing older can be a beautiful and normal part of life's cycle. We believe our bodies are designed and constructed for activity at any age. Fitness is truly ageless. You are exactly the right age to begin. Don't say you're too old to exercise. You're actually too old, regardless of your age, not to exercise.

The exercises and activities we suggest are for ordinary men and women—beginners—who are interested in health and wholeness. Start where you are, with what you can do, regardless of how little that is. Do not compare yourself with others but choose your own program; walk

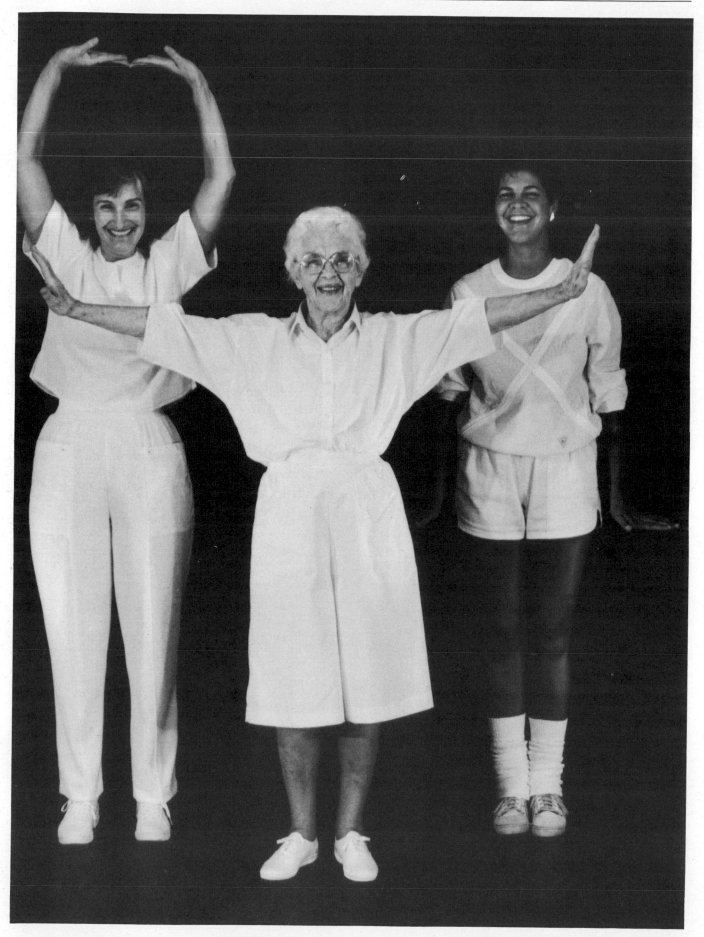

your own mile. Set your own goals that meet your needs and reflect your physical condition and objectives.

Most of us will never look like those trim, agile women or athletic, muscular men on the front covers of popular exercise manuals. It is easier to put on weight and harder to get it off as we get older. Wrinkles appear, shapes shift and change, sleep patterns may alter, activities may take more effort and be more limited, but older is beautiful, too! Our bodies are fortunate, not unfortunate, necessities and should be cared for as the amazing and precious gifts that they are.

We all count the number of days and years we live in the same way; however, the actual physical aging of our bodies during that count can vary as much as thirty years![1]

For example, you may be in your 50s but your internal physical system could be either that of a 65-year-old or a 35-year-old. Admittedly there are many things which contribute to longevity, including the potential for fitness and long life we inherit from our parents. For example, Grandma's mother, Lydia Miller, lived to be 97 years old. She went out fishing in a little rowboat on Shipshewana (Indiana) Lake well into her 80s—until the family felt she should not be out on the lake alone. Grandma's sister Gladys, who is almost 90, still walks two miles a day. So the potential in our family for fitness and longevity is positive. But the choices we make regarding lifestyle, habits, activity, nutrition, and rest all contribute to greater life expectancy.

Beth:

Someone once said, "Old age is always about fifteen years in the future." That someone could have easily been my grandmother.

Grandma Kauffman exemplifies all that I want to be when I am older. She has a remarkable mind and body, and her conviction that exercise must be a part of her life has certainly contributed to this. It is this particular conviction which keeps her young, but credit must also be given to her rare sense of humor in looking at herself, others, and everyday situations.

I remember when I first discovered the extent to which Grandma was exercising. Lori, my cousin, and I often went to visit Grandma while we were both students at Goshen College (the college which Grandma attended and from

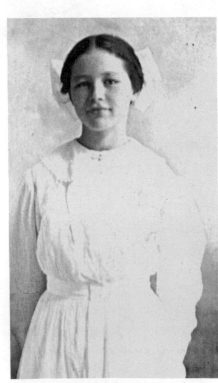

Nona, high school graduation, 1918 —age 19.

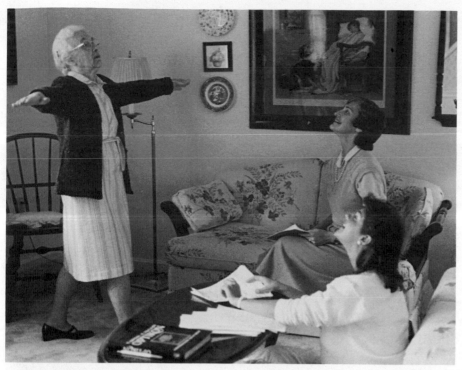

which Mom and I graduated). She lives at Greencroft, a lovely retirement center a few blocks from the college. One time she demonstrated her morning routine for us, and as we watched closely, we tried to control our laughter.

She began by lightly tapping all over her face with her fingers to stimulate the circulation in her face. Then she opened her eyes very wide and looked from one end of the room to the other. She became animated at this point, bending her knees slightly and holding out her arms. All she needed was a trench coat and hat to look like a detective creeping up on someone, looking ominously to the left and then to the right. Soon she was saying her ABCs with notable enunciation, and her face became fixed with a variety of interesting and unusual expressions. The best was yet to come, though.

The most hilarious display came when she showed us how she ran around her tiny apartment. She first darted over to the window, came to a screeching halt, peered both ways out the window, then catapulted across the room back into the bedroom. Lori and I couldn't stop laughing as she came flying out of the bedroom a few seconds later in a magniloquent jogging position. We all sat down and just laughed and laughed for a few minutes. Then she pointedly said to us, "You see, girls, I have to run, run, run, just to stay where I'm at."

My grandmother has definitely stayed "where she's at."

On my 13th birthday, my father took me riding and showed me how to drive a new Model T Ford. I can still remember the excitement! And it had no self-starter, only a "crank." Remember?
— Grandma

She has done this by exercising, maintaining a sense of humor, and being closely linked to the resources of family, friends, and church. I think these are the keys to her success, and it is important to remember this as you read our book. Not everyone is strikingly beautiful or has a body which could sell posters; however, we can all try to be as healthy as possible and be beautiful inside. It is imperative that I accept myself as I am, and part of this acceptance comes in being able to find humor in all aspects of life.

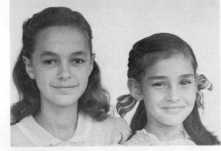

Naomi (right) and older sister Miriam, 1941—ages 9 and 12.

Naomi:

Mama has always been an energetic woman. Daddy, a more reserved person, loved that sparkle and excitement about her. As our family continues to experience her enthusiasm for life, we are learning from her how to grow older with grace, dignity, and gratitude.

When I was ten, my older sister Mim and I were walking home with Mama after a visit with a neighbor. Now there were not really hills in that little Texas town, but to us children it seemed that way. If you were riding a bike, you had to pump to get up to our house from Sara Unzicker's. As we walked, Mama looked over at us with a teasing face and a challenge in her voice and said, "I'll race you both up to the house!" Without another word we all three broke into a run. Mim and I ran as hard as we could but she got there first and sat down on the porch step, laughing, as though she had been there waiting for us. She was then 44. My younger sister, Judy, was born when Mama was 45.

Grandma:

"The longest journey begins with the first step."

After the death of my husband in 1977, I resolved that life must go on, and that the quality of my life would be just what I make it to be, joyous and rewarding or depressed and defeated.

It is an adjustment that only those who have lost a spouse or had a similar experience can understand. It is not a matter of trying to erase the memories, but rather of making them serve as a new dedication to an on-going life. Even with positive initiative, and constantly renewed courage and determination, there are periods of seeming failure. But I make a conscious effort to be optimistic and open-minded, to see the good in life, endeavoring to make a daily contribution in some way.

My daily gratitude for the goodness of God and the kind support of my entire family cannot be here adequately expressed. It has been uplifting, comforting, and reassuring. My hope is that my suggestions may be helpful to you, whatever your age and whether you are male or female.

Beth and Naomi:

As we have watched Grandma, we have discovered something important. She has made some very deliberate choices about how she will live. These have included staying physically active. Without consulting exercise manuals or books on how to slow the aging process, she has chosen to exercise vigorously and regularly. She has dispelled the myth that loss of strength and energy is necessarily due to getting older. It may simply be a lack of activity.

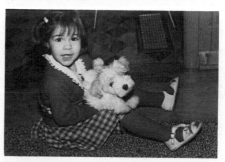

Beth, 1963—age 2.

"It was the best of times, it was the worst of times," wrote Charles Dickens long ago. A great part of the "best of times" has to do with our choices as we grow older. The more you choose to do, the more you *can* do. You don't have to go further or faster or longer than anyone else to feel successful. What matters is that you begin!

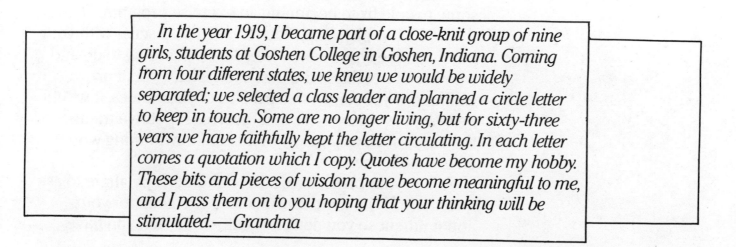

In the year 1919, I became part of a close-knit group of nine girls, students at Goshen College in Goshen, Indiana. Coming from four different states, we knew we would be widely separated; we selected a class leader and planned a circle letter to keep in touch. Some are no longer living, but for sixty-three years we have faithfully kept the letter circulating. In each letter comes a quotation which I copy. Quotes have become my hobby. These bits and pieces of wisdom have become meaningful to me, and I pass them on to you hoping that your thinking will be stimulated.—Grandma

2 Begin at the Beginning

*"You are always at the right age to make a
new beginning."*

If you have gotten this far you are at least considering starting an exercise program for yourself or modifying the exercises you are currently doing. Before starting to exercise or before increasing your current level of exercise, there are some important first steps for you to take.

While exercise is good for all people, not all exercises are good for all people. The first place to start is to check with your physician. In general, people over the age of 40, who have not been participating in a regular exercise program, should have some evaluations and studies done prior to starting. These evaluations should include a physical exam, a urinalysis, blood count, cholesterol and triglyceride measurements, fasting blood sugar and possibly an electrocardiogram. Most experts recommend a stress electrocardiogram or exercise EKG for those over the age of 40 who are beginning an exercise program. This is somewhat controversial in the minds of other experts since they feel that exercise is so important and so natural that insisting that these types of tests be done may prevent some people from beginning an exercise program. Discuss this with your physician. You should also discuss with your physician the type of exercise you are planning to do and whether or not this is the best exercise for you. For example, if you have osteoarthritis of your knees, it would be best to avoid exercise that involves repetitive trauma to the knees such as jogging. In this case, swimming would be an excellent exercise.[2]

Follow your physician's advice and don't be afraid to ask questions. Write them down before you go in for your appointment so you don't forget them. When you have your physician's go-ahead about how much you can do above your current level of activity and how quickly you can increase this, you are ready to begin.

Although each of us may be at a different age and stage in life, we are growing older at the same rate! Our energy supply, regardless of age, is not unlimited and we must use it efficiently. You can hardly add exercising to your day without eliminating some other activity. It is a matter of choosing priorities, and being disciplined.

The exercises we are outlining are interrelated but are designed to concentrate primarily on four areas: balance, coordination, flexibility and building muscle tone. (See Chapter 7 for a discussion of aerobic exercises.)

Several suggestions may help you get started.
1. Make your beginning your own personal one. Do you find satisfaction and support by having another person exercise with you? Do you prefer exercising alone? You may want to begin a program yourself and tell your friends about it later. Other people benefit from the support of others with similar goals.

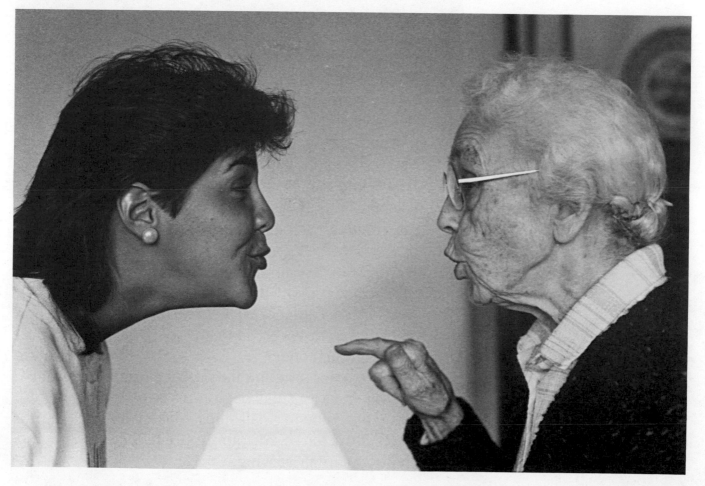

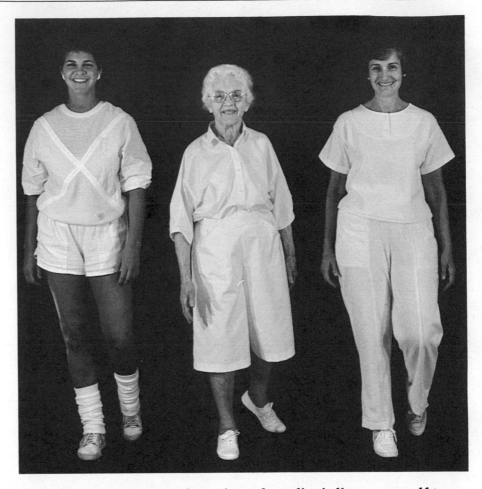

2. Choose a convenient time, but discipline yourself to a regular time. Notice in Chapter 4 what can be done before you get out of bed each morning. Some people like to exercise in the evening. A relaxing bath after your exercises is a good way to feel ready for sleep.

3. Set small, reasonable, achievable, measurable goals for yourself. Goals should be your own and not compared with those someone else may have. For example, your first goal may be: "I will do head, neck and shoulder exercises for three minutes, three times this week." It is reasonable and you can achieve it and measure the times you do it. Another might be: "I will walk one-half block three times this week." Good for you! It's a fine start and you can tell when you have accomplished it. Write down your goals and give yourself a gold star or some kind of reward when you have achieved each one.

4. Structure your program for success. Remember that what may seem like a small beginning is really a big step. Improvements come in small steps. Make your own chart or use a calendar to record your progress. It is encouraging to see how you are improving.

"Nothing worthwhile was ever accomplished without enthusiasm."

5. "No pain—no gain" is absolutely *not* true for older people and those who are interested in simple health maintenance. It may be true for younger athletes who are in serious training, but not for us. The limiting point for you should be a feeling of a bit more exertion than you would usually make, or a sense of tension in your muscles. Don't go much beyond that feeling at first. Your muscles may be a bit sore initially, but a good exercise program does not mean that you have to push to painful limits. You may want to alternate or switch exercises every other day to allow some of the muscles you may have stretched to recoup. It will gradually change as you continue to exercise regularly.

6. Listen to your body. It is a great source of information and monitoring. You can do this by taking your pulse rate or being aware of sensitive muscles when you are doing certain exercises. It can also be in the pleasure and "sync" which you and your body feel as you work together (see Chapter 7).

7. Be cautious if you experience pain, breathlessness, or discomfort of any sort from a certain exercise. Your body may be trying to tell you something. Persistent pain or discomfort may indicate you need to see a physician.

8. Take your time. Don't compare yourself with anyone but yourself and the progress you want to make. Be your own boss and set your own pace.

9. Write down the things which represent positive images of how an exercise program will benefit you. For example, imagine yourself walking a mile without being fatigued. Fresh air is going in and out of your lungs and you are feeling invigorated, alert, and energetic.

"I'm ready, willing, and able, but not all three at the same time."

It is enough to be ready and willing—the "able" will come with discipline and simply giving it a try.

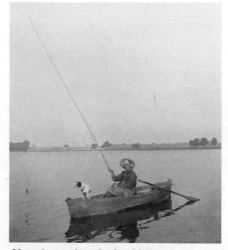

Nona's mother, Lydia Miller, fishing on Shipshewana (Indiana) Lake, 1949 —age 80.

17

3

Getting Off
to a Slow Start

*"Doing nothing is so tiresome.
You can't stop to rest."*

Whether you are starting at age 9 or 90, you can improve to a certain degree. Any increased activity is improvement. Exercises will vary greatly in their intensity and the demands they make on your body. You will want to start slowly.

For years, many Chinese people have begun their days by doing gentle, stretching, breathing, and joint exercises called Tai Chi. There are other exercises called Qi Gong designed for older persons with more fragile bones and joints. We can learn from them!

Spend a few minutes in simple, stretching, warm-up activities which can be incorporated into your daily morning routine. Use your own tailor-made Qi Gong. When you are first up in the morning and feel like yawning, do it with pleasure. Make it a long, loud, enjoyable yawn. If you feel like stretching, do it as long, leisurely, and luxuriously as possible. Move everything that feels like it needs to be stretched. Take some deep breaths that you can feel way down in your abdomen.

Put some energy into your movements as you bathe, shampoo and dry yourself. Be sure you have a tub mat to prevent slipping. You can roll up your towel and grab it at both ends, stretching it as far as you can. Hold it taut for a few seconds. Create your own routine, using the towel as a prop. Turn your body at the waist, bend over, then you can raise your arms above your head—still holding onto the towel.

You may prefer doing some warm-up exercises other than these suggested. Use exercises similar to the ones you will be doing later, only more limited and less vigorous. If you start out too vigorously, you can actually cause muscles to knot and be painful, as well as limit your flexibility later.

Try some of these to warm up:

1. Move your head forward and then back; then from side to side. *Move gently*. Do not snap or jerk.
2. Move your shoulders up and down a few times.
3. Move your arms up and down and flap like a bird a few times. Extend your arms and turn your hands in circles at the wrists; open and close hands.
4. Put your hands on your hips and turn at the waist from side to side.
5. Walk or run slowly in place for about a minute.
6. Take some deep breaths by inhaling as you raise your arms and dropping them as you exhale through your mouth. Then blow all the air out of your lungs.

These warm-up activities are important. You do not want to force your heart to work too hard, too soon. Your circulatory system needs time to supply sufficient blood to your heart as you get into more active exercises (see Chapter 7). This is especially true for beginners. Don't hold your breath. Begin to feel your breathing in rhythm with your motions.

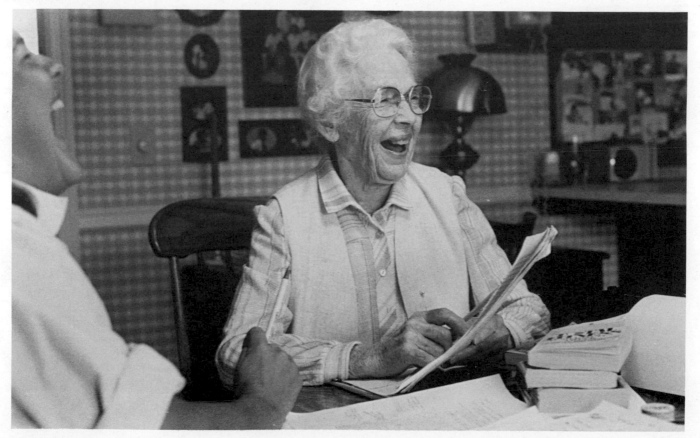

Wear lightweight, comfortable clothes. Underwear is fine. You are interested in exercising your muscles and not your temperature control. Overheating is not your goal and it does not necessarily mean that you're doing well because you've worked up a sweat. It may mean you are dressed too warmly. Drinking some water before or after your exercises will keep your fluid level at what it should be. Be aware of your need for water, especially when it is warm. □

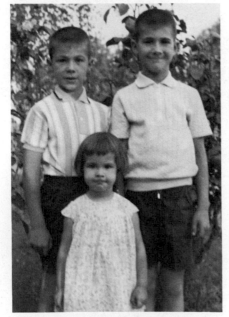

Philip (left), John Paul, and Beth Lederach—ages 6, 8, and 2.

Speaking of towels, Grandma says that although their family did not have a lot of money, they did have a lot of fun together. She recalls how she and her two sisters, Gladys and Ida, often had to wash and dry the dishes. Instead of being bored by these routine tasks, they made the work fun and played all sorts of games to keep things lively. One game was to throw their dish towels up in the air and see who could clap their hands the most number of times before catching the towel.

Another game was to start singing a song together when one of them had to leave to carry out the garbage. The point was to see if the person who left could come back singing the song and words at the same place as the persons who stayed.—Beth

Grandma's Chapter— Nona-Robics

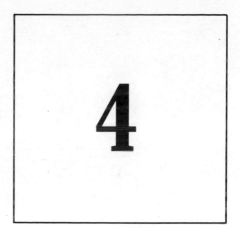

I live at Greencroft, a retirement home in Goshen, Indiana. Life here is pleasant, safe, and varied. Among the residents ranging in age from 60 to 100, there are many interesting people with different minds, personalities, talents, and opinions. There are abundant opportunities offered to those who still wish to be active and useful. Yes, we are very much alive here, although we move more slowly in body and mind. Sometimes amusingly so, like this—"Now, when I finally had it all together, I forgot where I put it," or "I simply can't walk all the way around this circle drive. I can make it half way; then I must turn around and go back," and, "I lost my keys, but I'm looking for my glasses." We can very sympathetically laugh with one another and that is good.

"A sense of humor is like a needle and thread; it can patch up a lot of things."

Now on to the exercises. I wish I could introduce them in a way that would greatly inspire you and put you into enthusiastic motion. You will find that this is what it takes if you wish to receive the possible benefits.

These are suggestions for ordinary people, in their 60s, 70s, and 80s, more or less. You need no fancy uniforms or expensive equipment. You can do them at home by yourself or with a friend, or in a small group without a leader.

They are not suggested because they are a cure for every ill, nor do I expect all of you to do each one just because someone else is able to do them, but I'm sure every effort will be rewarding. Since this is my own personal chapter, I may suggest exercises which are similar to those described elsewhere, but these are the ones I do each day.

You should first consult your doctor and then follow the

directions given. Don't do all the exercises the first day, but do some of them and don't put them off for the next morning (which never comes—it's always *this* morning!). Begin gradually; listen to what your body tells you. I find also that my body must listen to *me* sometimes when I say, "Oh, yes, you can do it. Try again!"

These exercises were not copied from a book or magazine or learned in an exercise class but are those that I tried from time to time and have found very helpful. Add some of your own.

Morning Exercises

You can begin even before you throw the covers back or sit up.

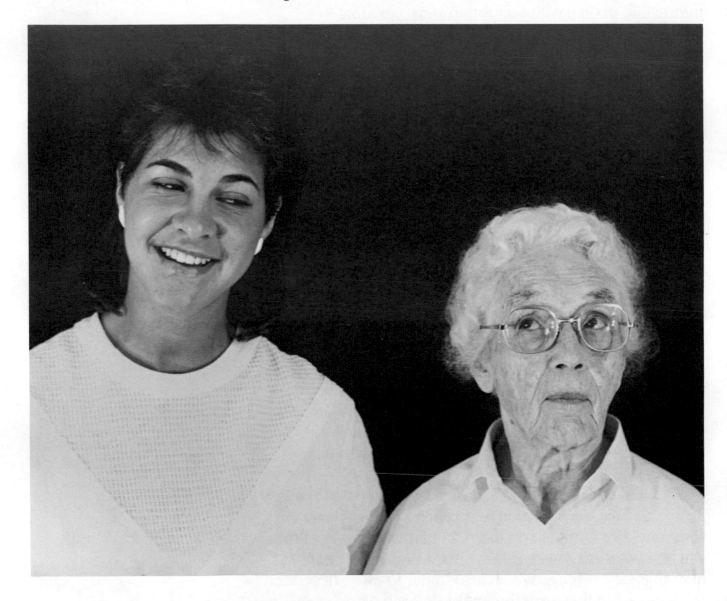

1. **Start at the top**

   A. Exercise your eyes and face. Roll your eyes from side to side, look up and down from the corner of the ceiling on your right to the floor on your left; reverse the motion.

   B. Open your eyes wide, then close them. Do this 10 times. While you are moving your eyes, you can be moving your face muscles from side to side.

   C. Move your jaw up, then back and forth.

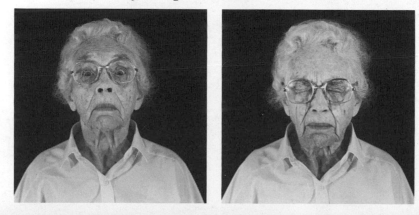

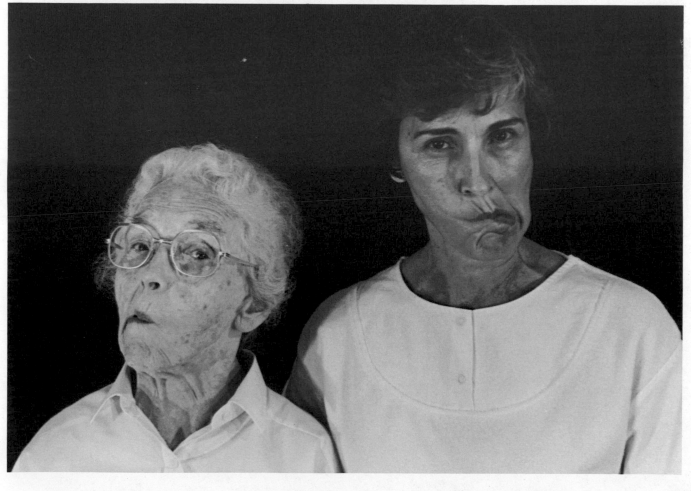

D. Greatly exaggerate the motions of your face and lips to say the vowels.

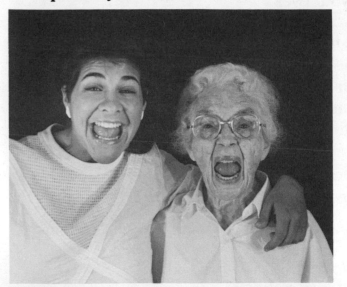
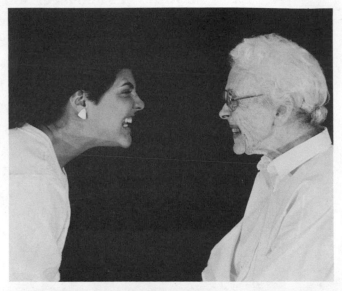

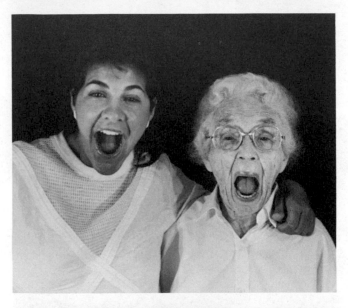
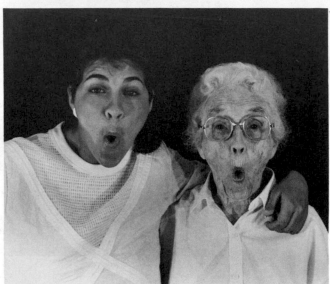

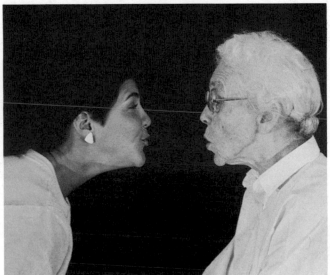

These exercises are stimulating and good for muscle tension and relaxation.

2. Now you are fully awake!

    A.   Sit up in bed and swing your arms from side to side, pulling the muscles in your hands and arms.

    B.   Stretch your legs and feet out straight and, without bending your knees, raise your arms above your head, then down to touch your toes. Count as you do these motions or you will declare you did them 20 times and it was really only 12.

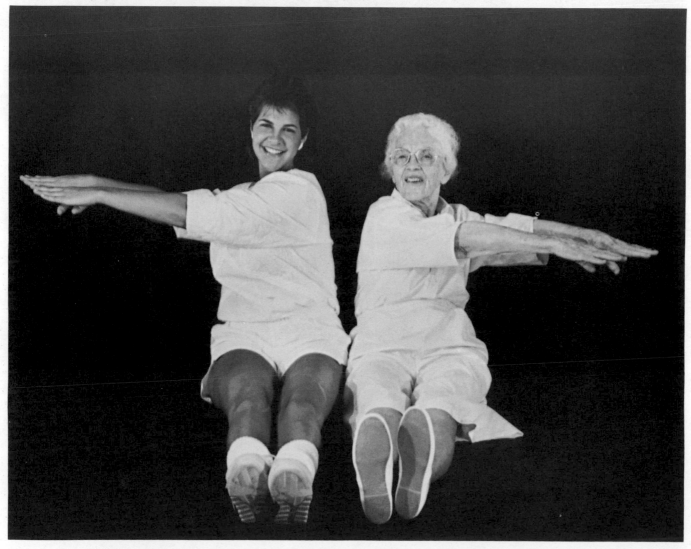

3. Next step:
    A. Lie down again.
    B. Stretch out your legs and without bending the left knee, raise your right foot. This may be difficult at first, but keep trying. Reverse the motion and count. Do it a few more times each morning. Now swing out of bed, landing firmly on both feet.

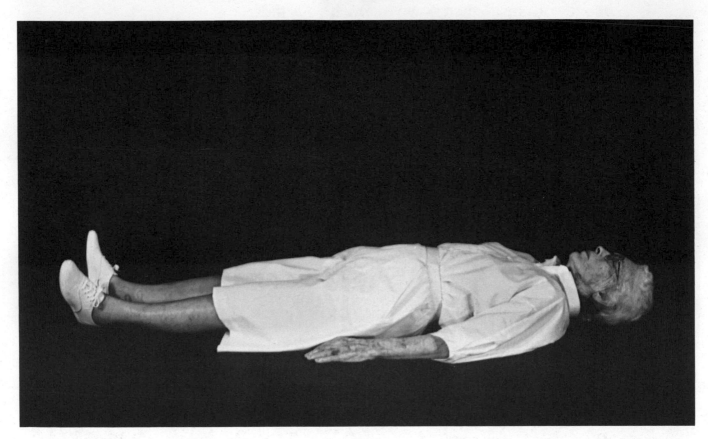

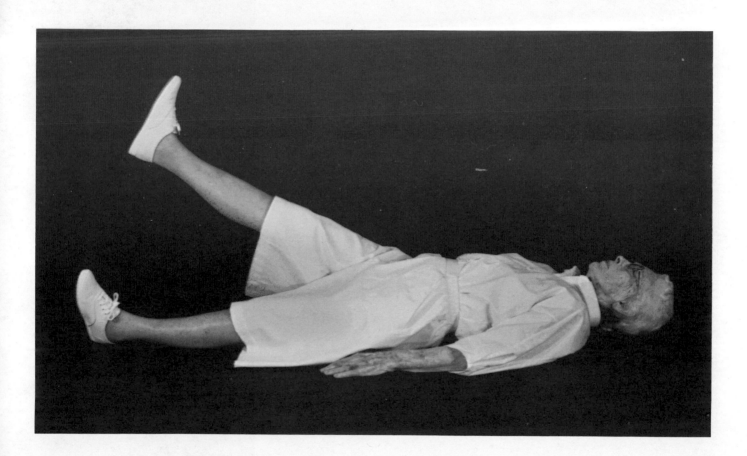

4. **Now that you're up:**
    A. Touch your hands behind your back (count 1).
    B. Touch them straight above your head (count 2).
    C. Extend your arms and touch your hands in front of you (count 3). Repeat.

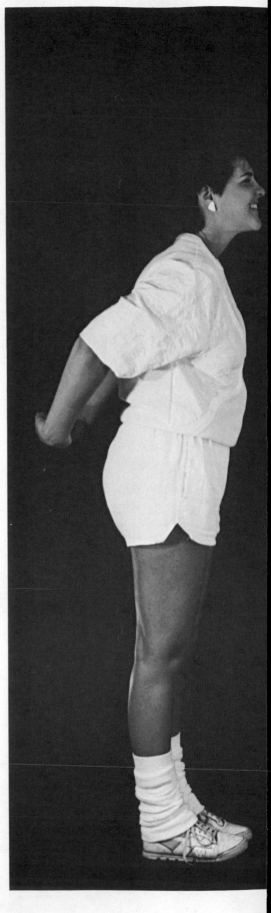

Make your words sweet today. Tomorrow you may have to eat them.

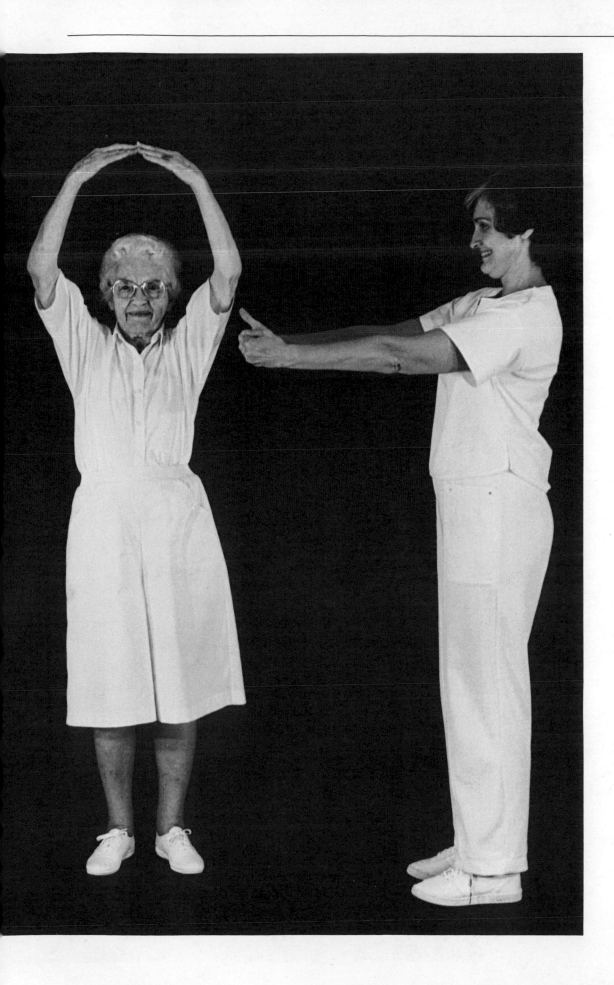

5. Stay flexible!
   A. Swing your right arm around your head in front and let your fingers clasp the back of your neck. Then do the left arm. Repeat.
   B. Now reach around the back of your head and clasp your hand around your neck. Do this with your other hand. Repeat.
   C. Swing your right arm over the top of your head, touching your left ear. Do it with your left arm touching your right ear.

You will be surprised how helpful these exercises can be and how they will help you with activities like combing your hair or dressing.

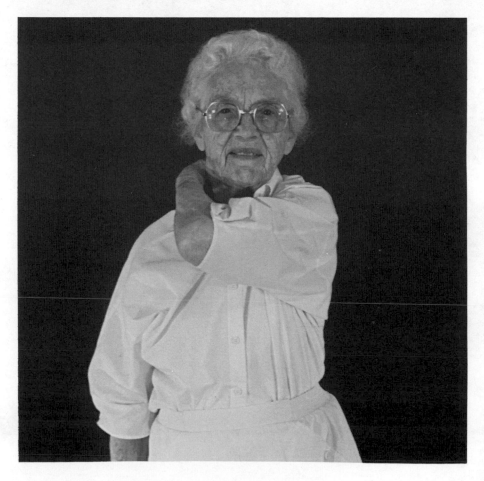

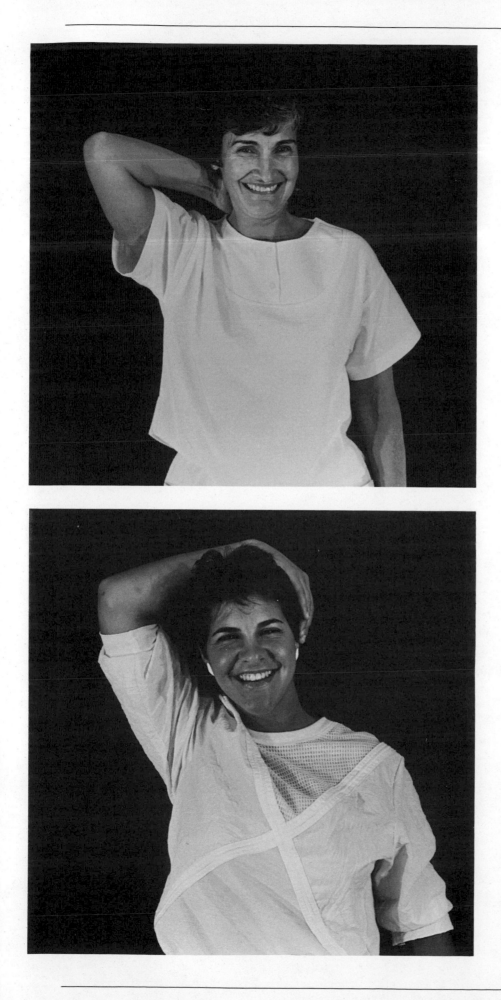

6. Now get your body moving:
   A. Hold both arms straight out in front.
   B. Turn your body and arms as far to the right as possible, then to the left. Repeat as you are able.

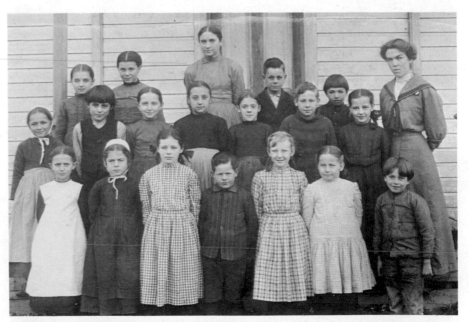

Naylor School, Middlebury, Indiana, 1911. Nona, age 12, is third from the left on the bottom row.

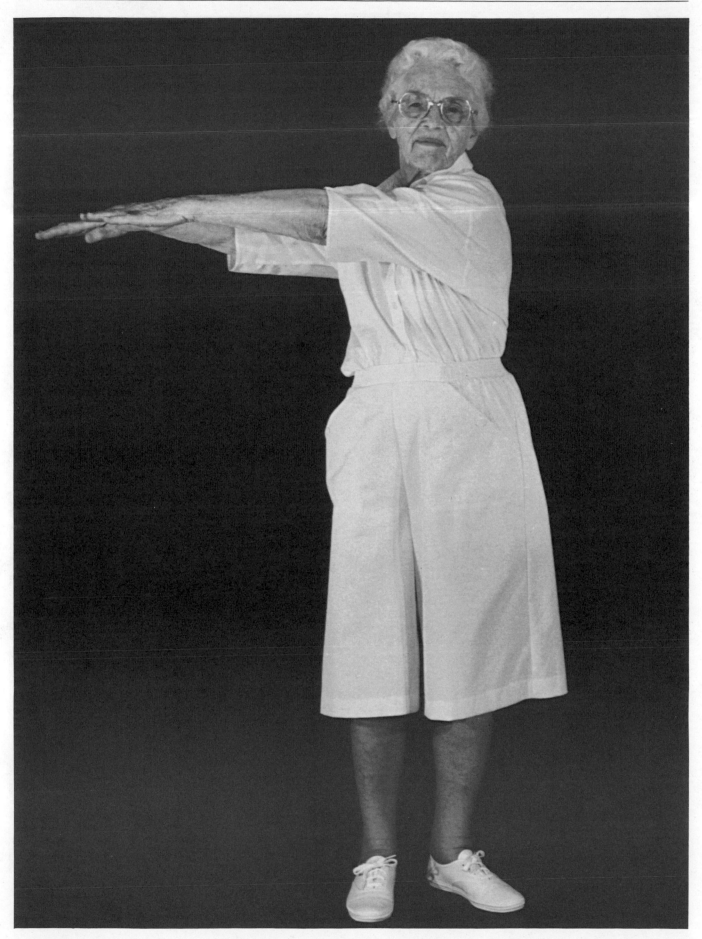

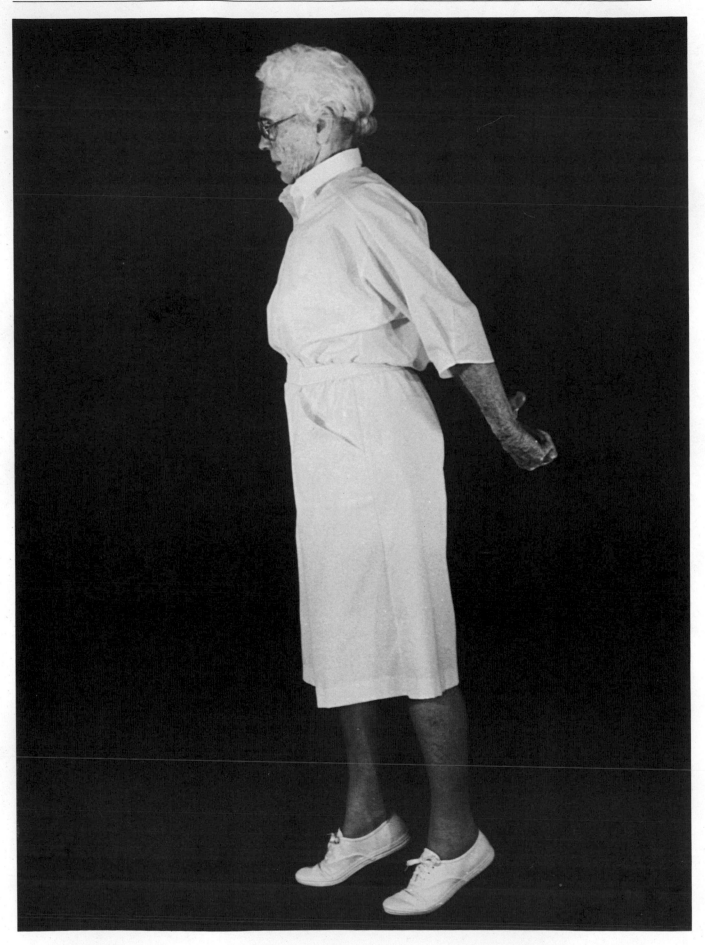

7. Walk on tiptoe:

    A.   Clasp your hands tightly behind you, stretching the muscles in your chest and lower body.

    B.   Walk on your toes if possible.

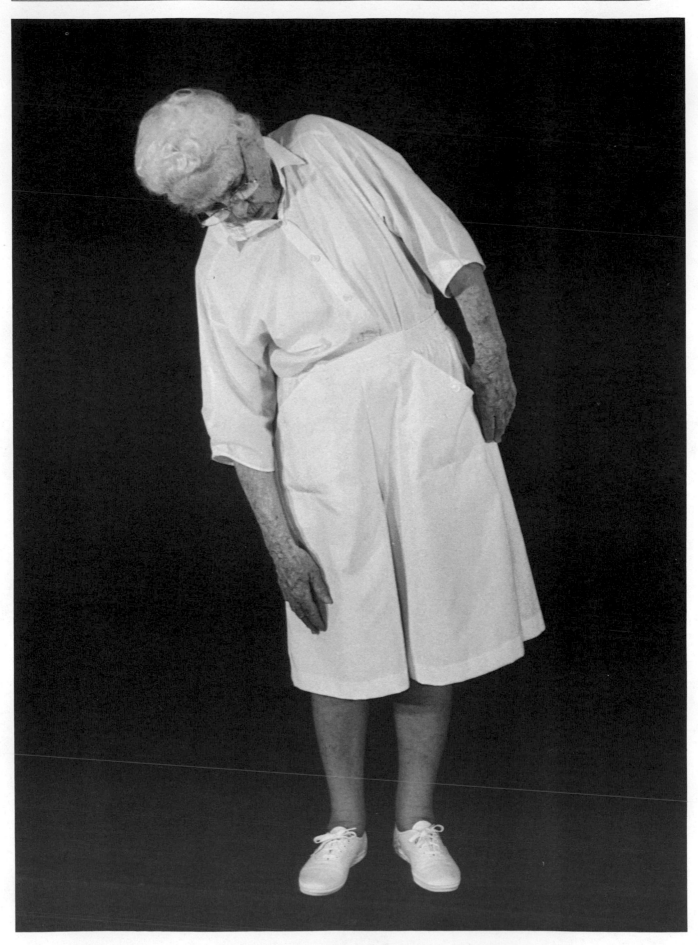

8. **Shoulder exercises:**
    A. Stand up straight.
    B. Now drop one shoulder; lift the other shoulder as far as possible, stretching the muscles down your back. You can even feel it pulling in your thigh and leg.
    C. Reverse the shoulder motion.

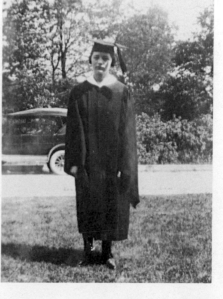

Nona, graduation from Bluffton (Ohio) College, 1925.

Grandma's father insisted that his daughters go to high school when it was not a very acceptable thing for girls to do. Grandma says she recalls him saying, "Girls, I want you to leave the world a better place than you found it, somehow, in some way and some place, and I think you can do that by going to high school." As it turned out, they all three also went to college and became teachers.—Beth

9. Slowly on this one!
   A. Stand straight without bending your knees.
   B. Touch your knees, ankles, and then the floor. To avoid any injury, do this slowly.

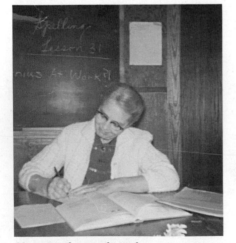

Nona as the teacher of a one-room school at Honeyville, near Topeka, Indiana, 1952.

Seldom in my life have I felt as helpless as I did when I entered a country schoolroom on my very first day of school teaching. Forty pupils, grades one to eight, all subjects, nine beginners who could not speak English, only German, and all eyes on the teacher. And all this for $2.50 a day. "I came, I saw, I conquered" and loved it.—Grandma

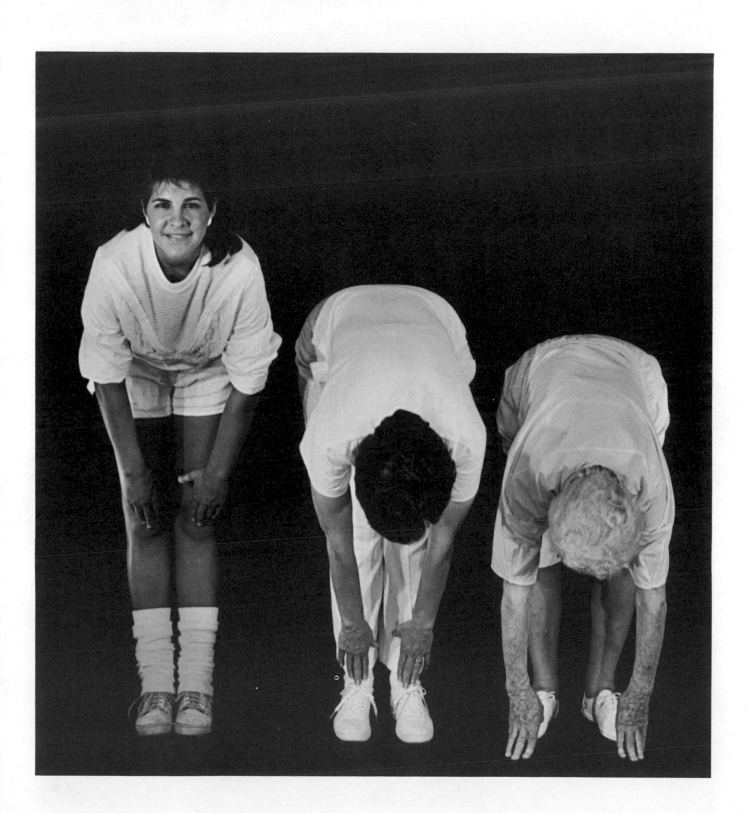

10. **Breathing exercises:**

I like to feel I am breathing fresh air so I go outside or open a window. Inhale slowly; through your nose, then exhale slowly, ending with a little cough so the air will be expelled. Repeat.

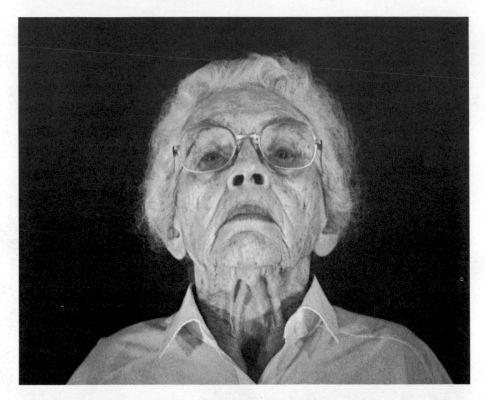

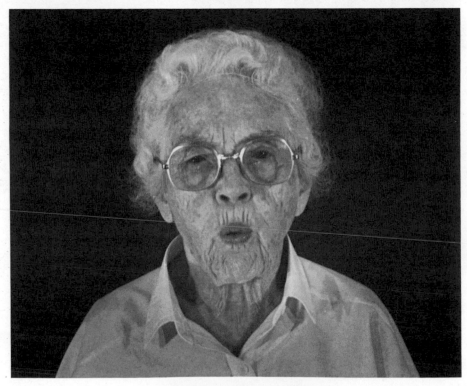

Walking

Walking is one of the best exercises you can do. If you walk briskly, swinging your arms as you walk, you use almost every muscle in your body. It gives you a feeling of well-being and vitality. It is a very good remedy for overweight, a lack of interest in life, a loss of energy and appetite. It has many times been found helpful for those with heart problems.

There are numerous examples of older people who have regained strength and renewed health by simple exercises and walking. I walk a mile or two every day and since I use a pedometer, I know that I have ticked off over 1000 miles.

You will find more information and helpful suggestions about walking in Chapter 7 of this book. If at all possible, do try it. You'll be pleased with what it does for you.

"You cannot make a peach out of a potato,"
but you can be improved!

Conclusion

To my dear senior friends, may you somehow live better and feel better because of the exercises recorded here. It would be a great pleasure to meet you. We have lived through the most rapidly changing times of all history. We have seen the first cars, telephones, electric appliances, TVs, radios, and even a man walking on the moon. There have been many changes in the variety and availability of foods, and in the fields of education and medicine. We have grown, changed, and survived. We want to keep on growing—without growth there is no life.

These exercises are really only part of the other exercises described in this book. I have learned to do many of them also and have experienced a real sense of accomplishment. You will feel like a winner if you learn to step, swing, bend, count and pull. Keep trying! "Practice makes perfect."

Personally, I am sustained by my faith in an eternal God, by my family and by lasting friendships, by my church, my interest in life and hope for tomorrow. My prayer is, "Lord, keep me alive as long as I live," be it in my own home, a retirement home or in a nursing home.

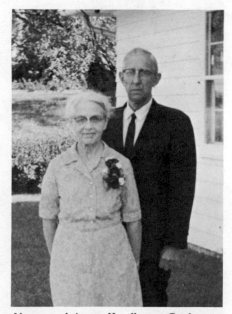

Nona and Amsa Kauffman, Goshen, Indiana, 1964.

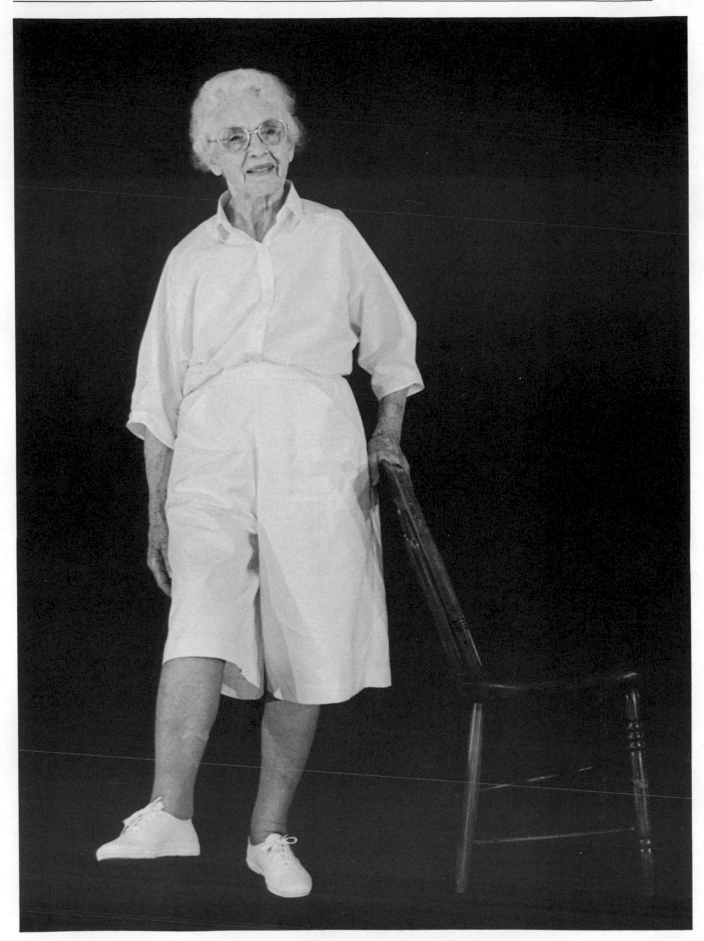

Coordination and Balance

*"The dictionary is the only place where you
find success before work."*

Sometimes when we have not been very active or have
limited mobility, it is difficult to coordinate movements. You
may discover that when you try to move your arms and
feet at the same time, they simply won't cooperate. This
difficulty with coordination is not necessarily a part of
aging, but may be because of apprehension about falling or
because you simply stopped trying certain activities that
require more coordination.[3] It may take a while to do some
of these exercises, but see how much you can improve with
practice. Don't be discouraged!

A simple exercise to practice getting your arms and legs
moving together is to walk in place and pretend you are
swimming with your arms. You may find that music with a
rhythm that fits the speed of your movements will help you
with coordination.

Try one or two of these until you feel you can do them
quite well before you move on to another one. It may take
a few days or weeks to do them smoothly. It is like learning
to sing a song or play the piano. Practice each note
(movement), one at a time. Then you can play the chords
(series of movements). Soon you will know the entire song
(complete exercise) and can sing or play it well!

Concentration is very important. Be sure to hold on to a
sturdy, armless chair with non-skid feet or something
stable, if it is hard to maintain your balance.

The following series of five exercises are for improving
your coordination but require balance as well.

1. HOP-SCOTCH

A. Stand with your feet about shoulder-width apart or until you feel you have a comfortable balance.

B. Now bring your arms up to the level of your shoulders and extend them straight out at your sides.

C. Bend your left knee and bring that left foot up. You will be standing on only one foot, so do it slowly and try to maintain your balance. Keep

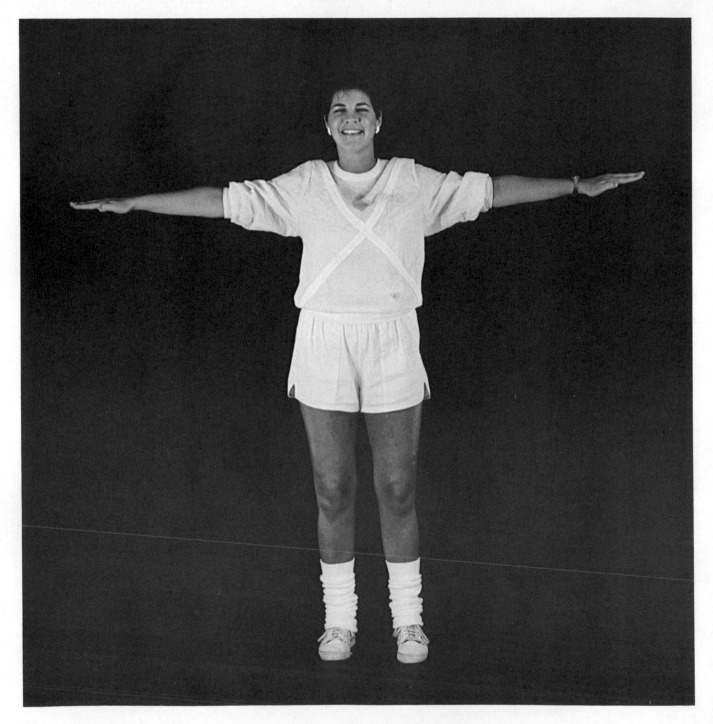

your back as straight as possible.

D. Slowly touch your right hand to your left toes. Then return to the starting position with your arms extended.

E. Repeat the sequence, only this time bring your right foot up and touch it with your left hand. Do these 10 times or so, until you feel a nice rhythm and can stand without holding on to anything.

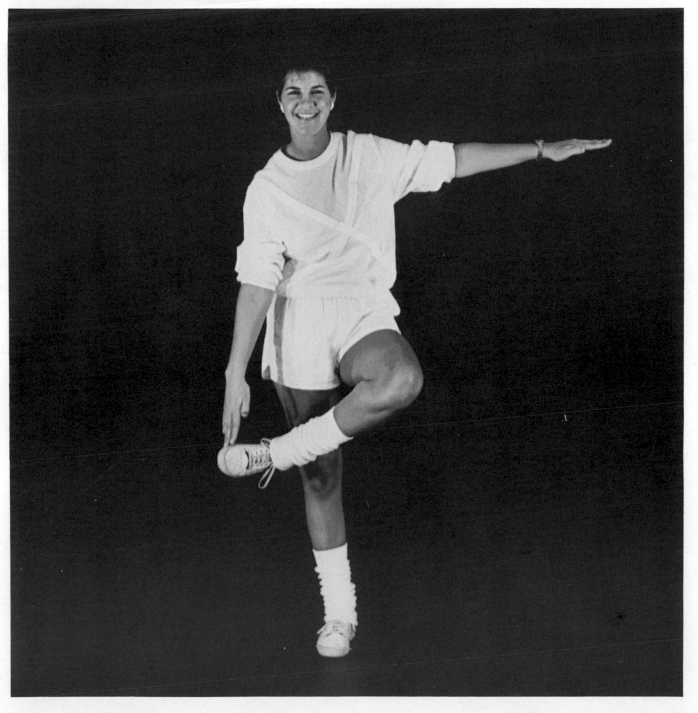

2. KNEE HIGHS

A. Stand with your feet apart in a comfortable position.

B. Bring your hands up to your shoulders and make fists.

C. Now bring your left knee up and move your right elbow down to touch your knee. You will be

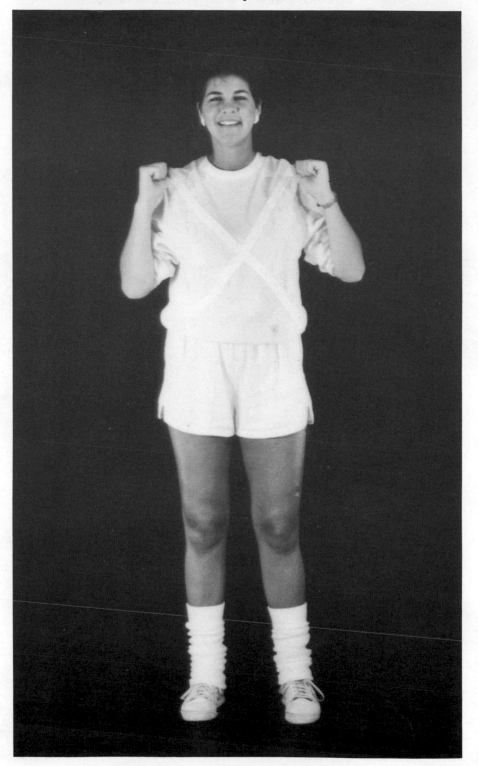

standing on one leg again, so be careful.

D. Return to the starting position and then repeat the sequence, bringing your right knee up and touch your left elbow. Concentrate and repeat the motions slowly until you can do them fairly smoothly and still keep your balance.

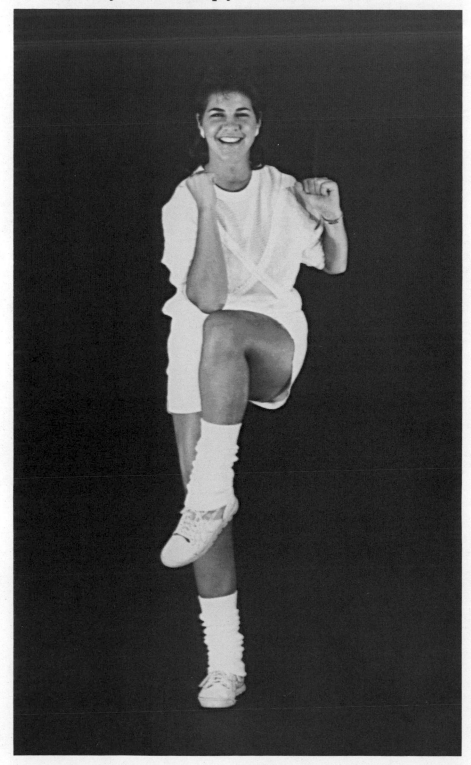

3. ARM SWINGS

A. Stand with your feet apart in a comfortable position.

B. Extend your left leg out in front of you, with your toe pointed, touching the floor with your toe.

C. At the same time, swing both arms down and to the left side of your body. Give your arms a hefty swing as you do this and twist a bit at the waist, too.

D. Return to the starting position and then repeat the same motions,

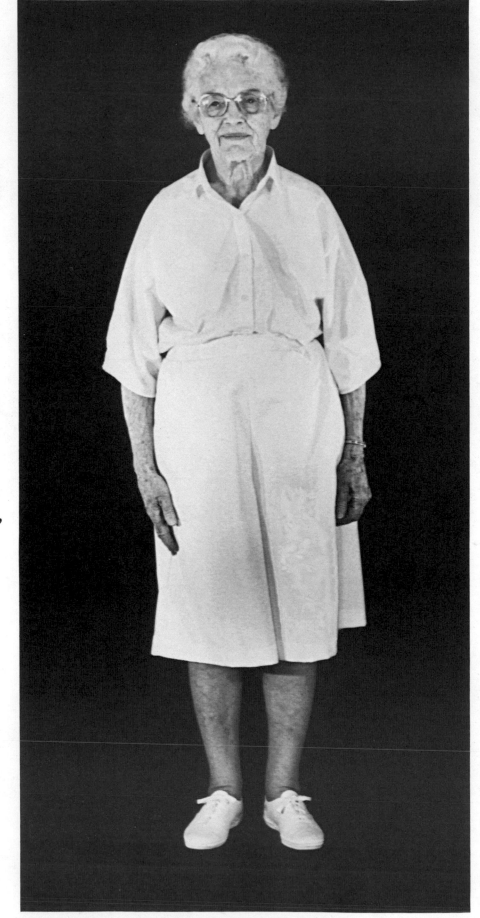

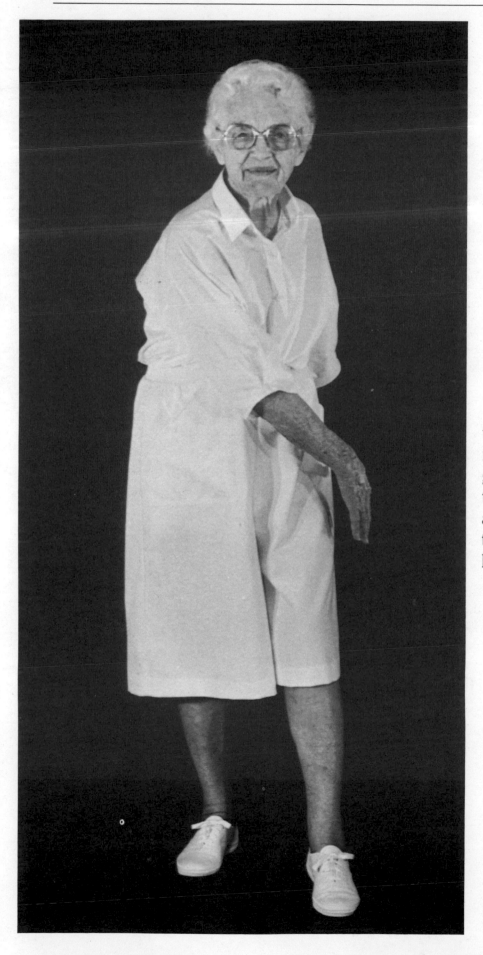

touching the floor with your right toe. Now swing your arms down and to the right side of your body, again twisting at the waist as you swing.

E. Alternate the motions, left—right—left—right—until you have a nice swinging rhythm going.

Giving yourself directions out loud with a little rhythm may help you get going smoothly. Say: "Left toe—touch floor—both arms—to/the/left." Doing this with music would help, too.

4. "POINT-SET-TOE"

A. Get in a comfortable standing position again, with feet about shoulder-width apart.

B. Keep your elbows at your waist and raise your hands to your shoulders with palms facing forward.

C. With left toes pointed, swing left leg forward and touch floor with toes.

D. At the same time (and this is the tricky part!) extend your right arm fully, straight forward, palm down. Then return to starting position.

E. Now repeat the motions with right leg, toes and arms.

This one takes a bit more concentration because it seems easier to move either right arm and right leg or left arm and left leg *together* rather than as opposites! Say the directions out loud and move slowly. You will get it!

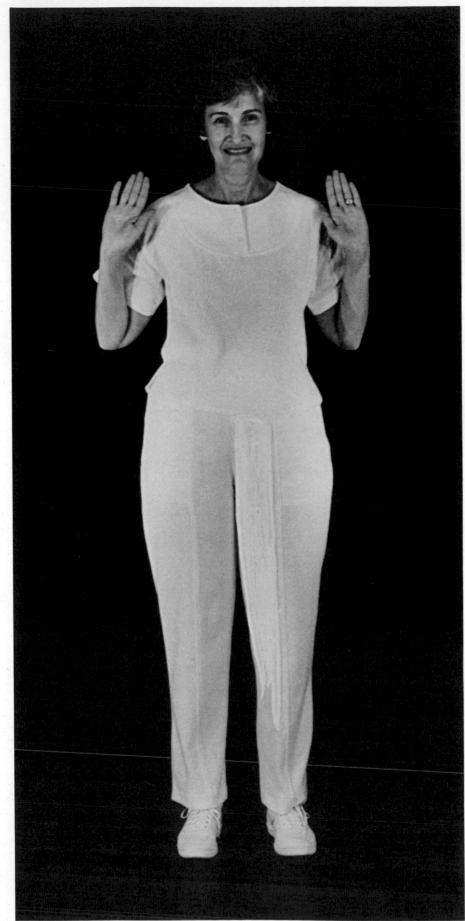

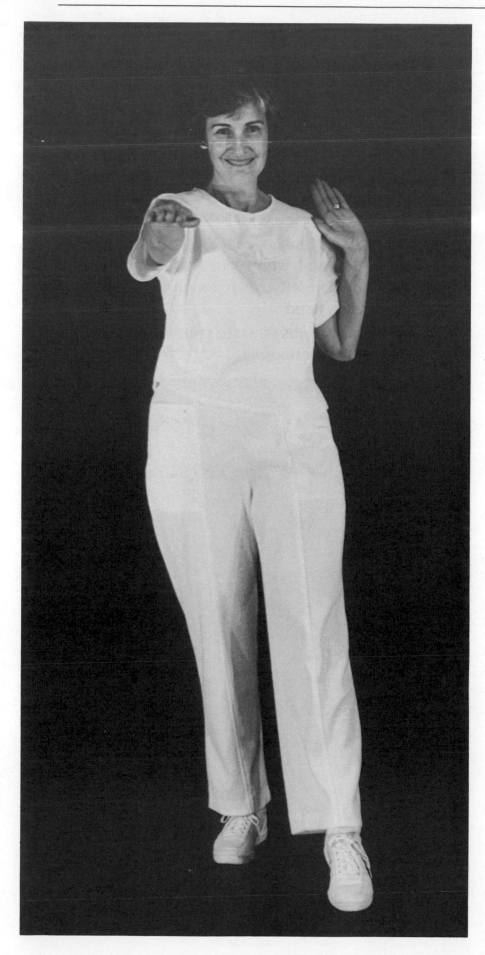

Recently at a banquet for retired people, Grandma received recognition for having driven a car the most number of years. She also "stood" the longest and won a spelling bee at her retirement home. The word that finally stumped her (and the audience as well!) was "idiosyncracy."—Beth

5. NOSE TO EARS TOUCH

This exercise is mostly for fun but is nevertheless quite a challenge!

A. Stand in a comfortable position with your hands on your thighs.

B. With your right hand, touch your nose. At the same time (left arm crossing over right arm) touch your right ear with your left hand.

C. Bring your arms down to your thighs again.

D. Now do just the opposite! Touch your nose with your left hand, while your right arm crosses in front of your left arm, to touch your left ear with your right hand.

E. Bring your arms down to your thighs again and repeat the motions.

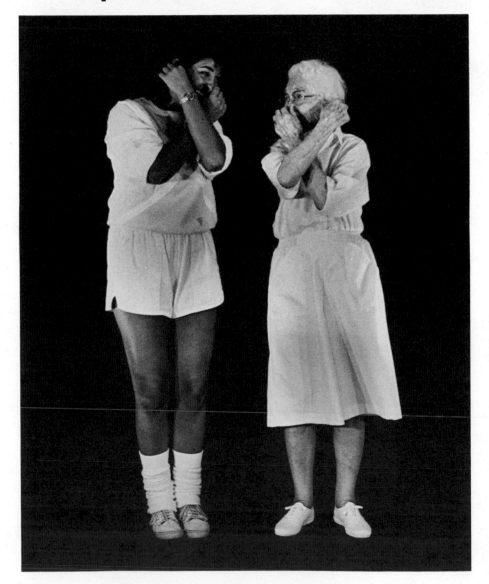

This is really more difficult than it looks! It takes quite a bit of concentration and practice. You will amaze your family and friends if you can get this one going. Just ask them to try if they think it looks easy.

Remember with all these exercises to be aware of whether you feel you have mastered them and can do them smoothly. The number of times we suggest doing each one is only a guide. Remember that "every man must do his own growing no matter how tall his grandfather was."

"Stand aside and watch yourself go by."

Have you looked at yourself in a full-length mirror lately? Take time to do that now. Look at yourself from all sides. Do you hold your head high? Are your shoulders held up and back? What about your abdomen?

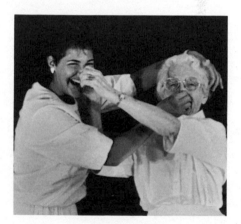

As you work through these rather simple exercises that are designed to help you with balance, you will also develop a sense of confidence and grace that comes from knowing you have good posture. Make an effort as you try these to improve the tone of your abdominal muscles as well. Lift your chest a bit, let your shoulders fall back and down to a comfortable position, and pull your abdomen in and up and hold it. Does that look better?

It is not uncommon for the abdomen to be larger than it used to be. It may be from fat accumulation, from loss of muscle tone or from poor posture. But there is also the possibility that as you age, the vertebrae in the spinal column get smaller and the spine may actually be shortened. Your ribs, in turn, get closer to your hips and the abdominal organs must go somewhere. So the abdomen expands and you begin to be aware of the need to pull in your stomach.

Some exercises which work at strengthening abdominal muscles may cause injury to your vertebrae if they are particularly fragile. Be sure to check with your doctor for a program especially suitable for you. Simply standing up as straight as you can, pulling in your abdominal muscles as tightly as you can and holding that position for 10–15 seconds, may help. Tense these muscles, then relax. You can do this anytime, sitting or standing, as often as you like or whenever you think about it.

The following exercises are designed to help improve your balance, and keep you flexible as well. It is a good idea to hold onto a chair with one hand. Be sure the chair is pushed up against a wall so it won't scoot away. As your balance improves, you may be able to do these without the chair. Again, try one or two for a few days until you feel you are ready to try another one.

6. "REMARCHABLE"

A. Raise your right knee as high as possible, as though you are marching.

B. Then return to starting position again.

C. Now lift your left knee as high as possible and repeat: right knee, left knee, right knee. Do this until you feel some muscle resistance or tension as you raise your knee higher. You may want to count just to see if you are able to do more and lift your knee a bit higher as you do these from week to week. This improves the muscle tone in your legs and your abdomen.

"Don't complain about being old—it is a privilege denied to many."

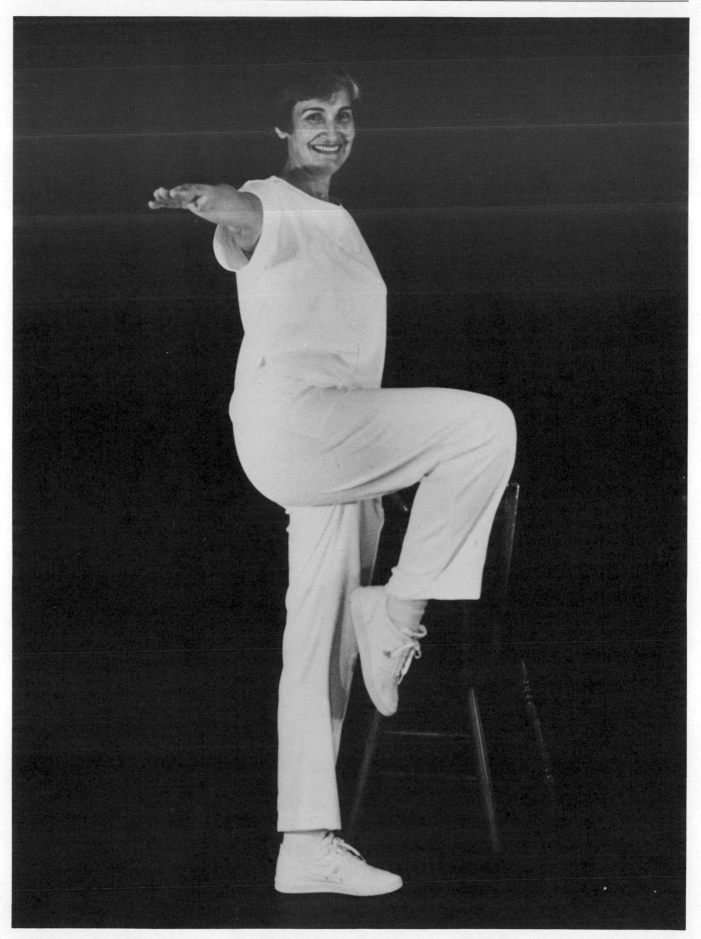

7. "MAKING TRACKS"

A. Pretend you are trying to walk on a railroad track. Find a line on the floor covering or carpeting or put a piece of string in a straight line across the floor.

B. Extend your arms and raise them about as high as your shoulders to help you keep your balance.

C. Begin to walk, placing one foot *directly* in front of the other one, following the line you have made.

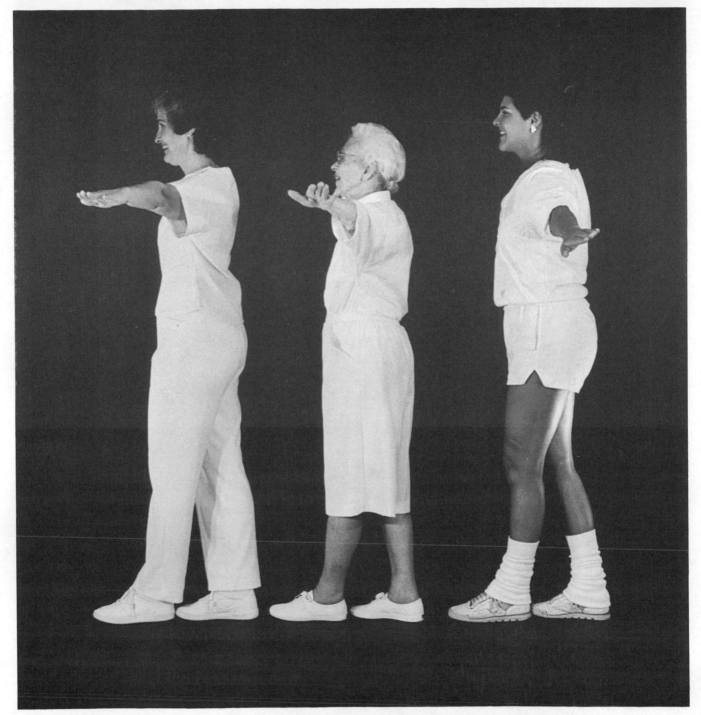

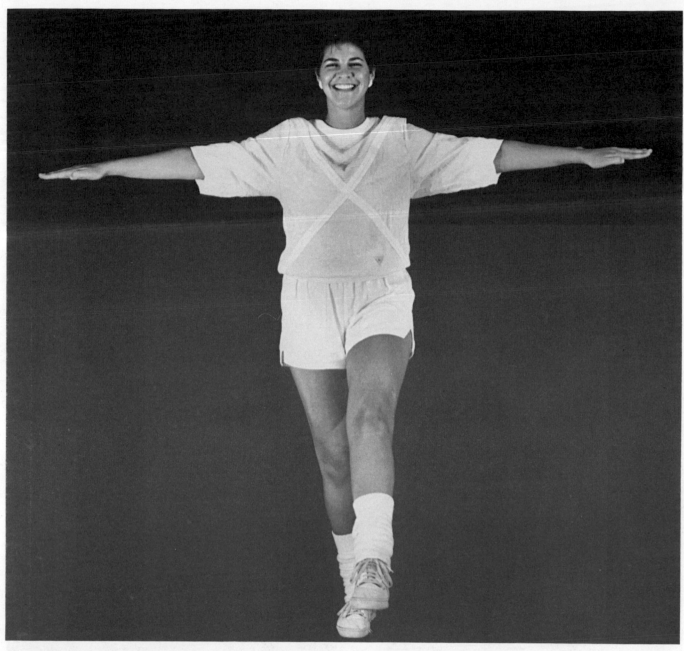

8. ONE-LEG STAND

Although this may sound and look rather simple, it is a bit more difficult. Hold on to something to maintain your balance if necessary.

A. Start with your feet planted firmly and comfortably on the floor.

B. Extend arms and lift them to shoulder height.

C. Swing left leg out and up in front of you without touching the floor and hold it as you count to five.

D. Repeat this with the right leg. Try to keep your body as motionless as possible when your leg is extended.

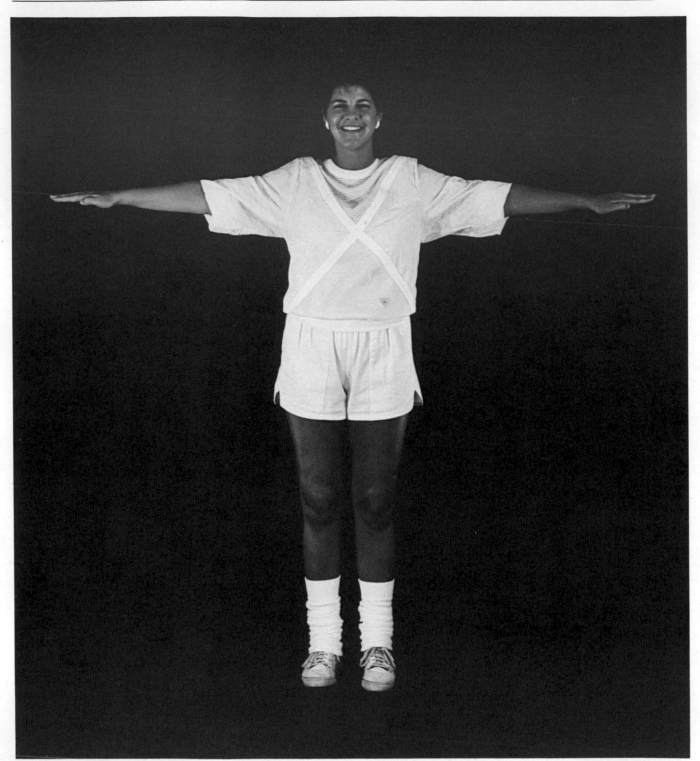

9. "SWING-SHIFT"

    A.   Stand with feet apart in a comfortable position.

    B.   Lift and extend your arms to shoulder height.

    C.   Now swing left leg to the side of your body, with toe pointed, and hold for five counts.

    D.   Return to starting position and then repeat the motion with your right leg.

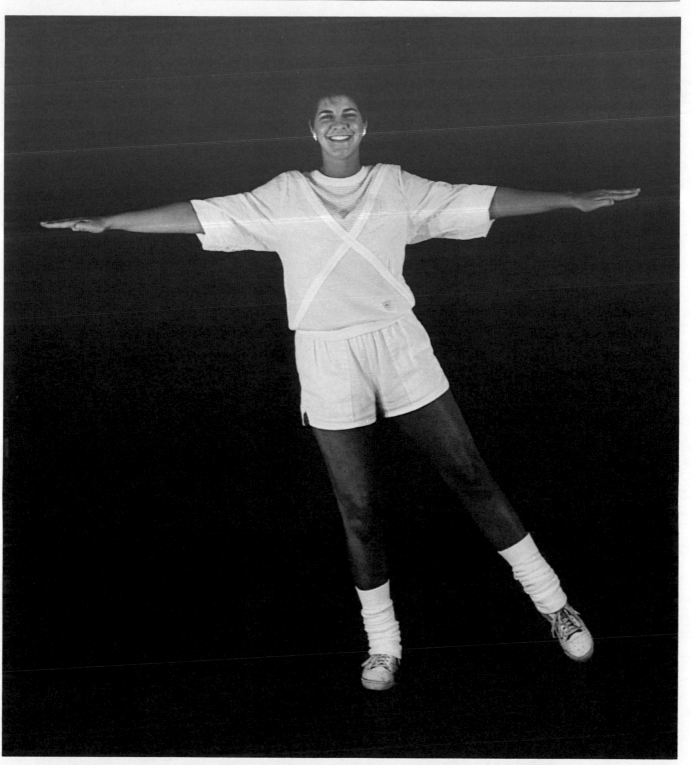

E.   A variation of this would be to swing your leg out
     and up in front of you as in the previous exercise,
     but instead of putting your foot back on the floor,
     swing your leg to the side of your body in one
     continuous motion.

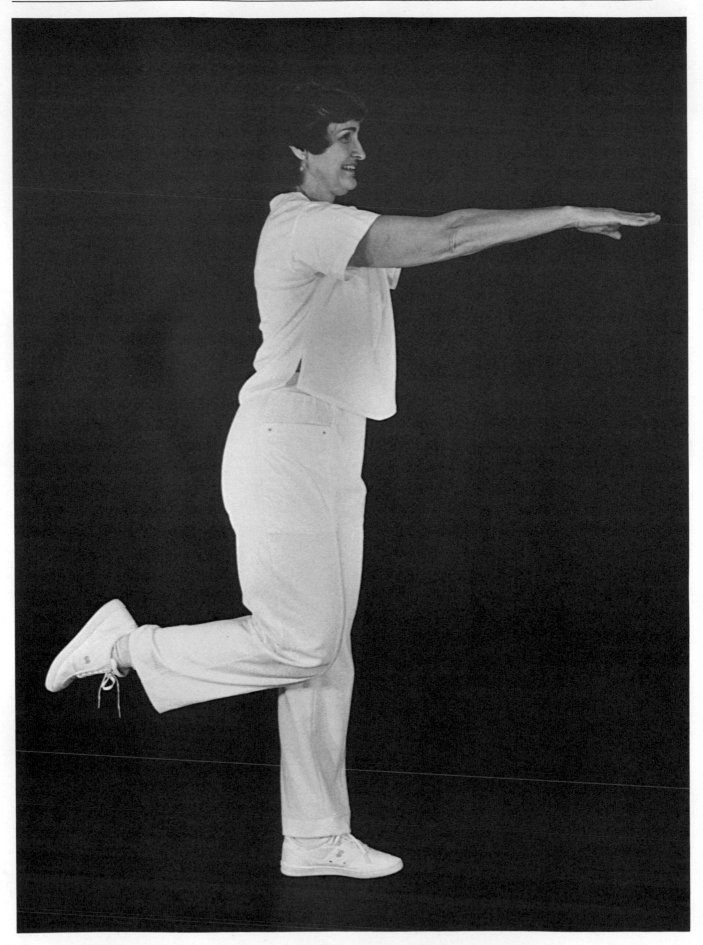

10. "REARS AND TOE TUCK" (Just like you ordered from the catalog!)

    A.   Place your feet in a comfortable standing position.

    B.   Extend your arms straight out in front of you.

    C.   Stand on your left leg, with your right leg bent at the knee, and your heel up toward your buttocks. Hold that position for five counts.

    D.   Return to starting position and then repeat the motion with your right leg.

As you practice these exercises that can help you with improving coordination and balance, you are also working at keeping your body flexible. These exercises help to increase your circulation, too. You should experience more confidence and poise when you feel your balance and posture has improved. Look in the mirror and see if you can tell a difference!   ☐

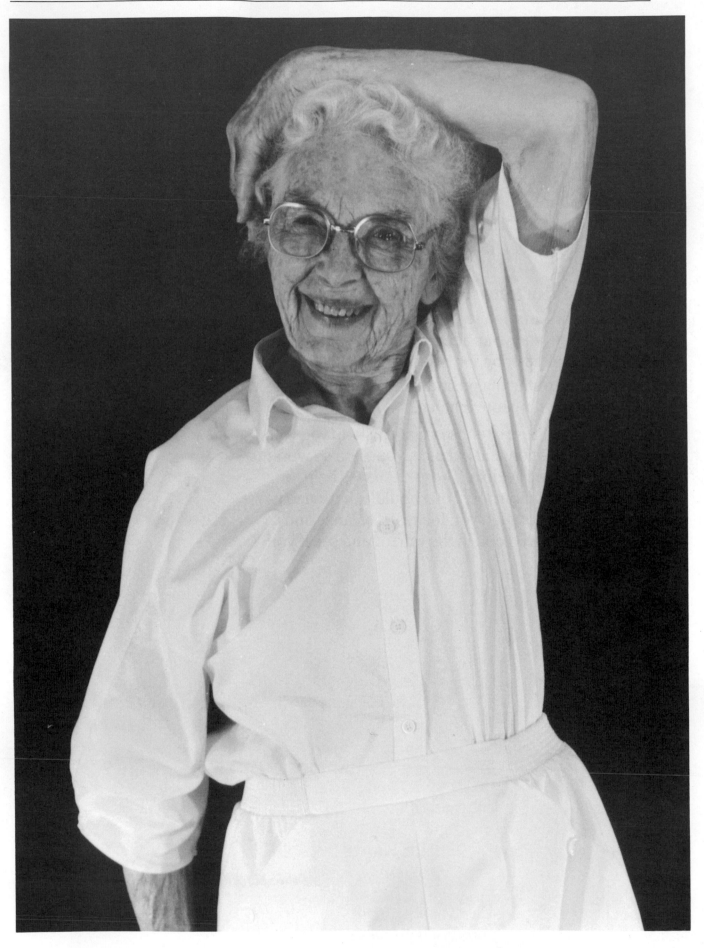

Take It From the Top

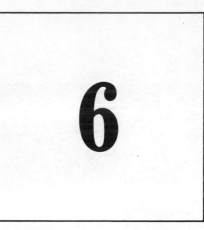

"You can't gain energy by saving it. You can only gain energy by spending it."

The more you use your body, the better it works. It is nourished by exercise. Each group of muscles needs to have a work-out. Exercises that allow more steady movement of many muscles and do not involve highly stressful exertion are best. Maintaining mobility, flexibility, or a full range of motion in all joints is a primary goal. But muscle tone is enhanced and muscle mass is also built as you work at fitness. Again, concentrate on one or two exercises or motions until you feel you can do them with some ease, yet feel some exertion or tension as you move.

These exercises are most effective when you are standing but may also be done while seated on a chair if you are unable to stand. If you need to hold onto a chair, be certain it is placed firmly against a wall so it will not scoot.

Sometimes we are hardly aware that we are tense. Very often this shows up in the neck and shoulder area. You cannot really eliminate this tension unless you become aware of it first. Although the next exercises are designed primarily to help maintain flexibility, they are great for relieving tension or stiffness which can so easily occur.

The human head is actually quite heavy for the neck to hold and turn from side to side! If you sit at a desk, or in one position doing hand-work for a length of time, there is a strain placed on the neck and shoulder muscles. If you stop for a bit and do a few of the following exercises, it will help eliminate that pain in your neck, upper back and shoulders. Bird-watching can be done more comfortably, too, if you keep these muscles flexible. Begin very slowly and gently. Speed is not important with these.

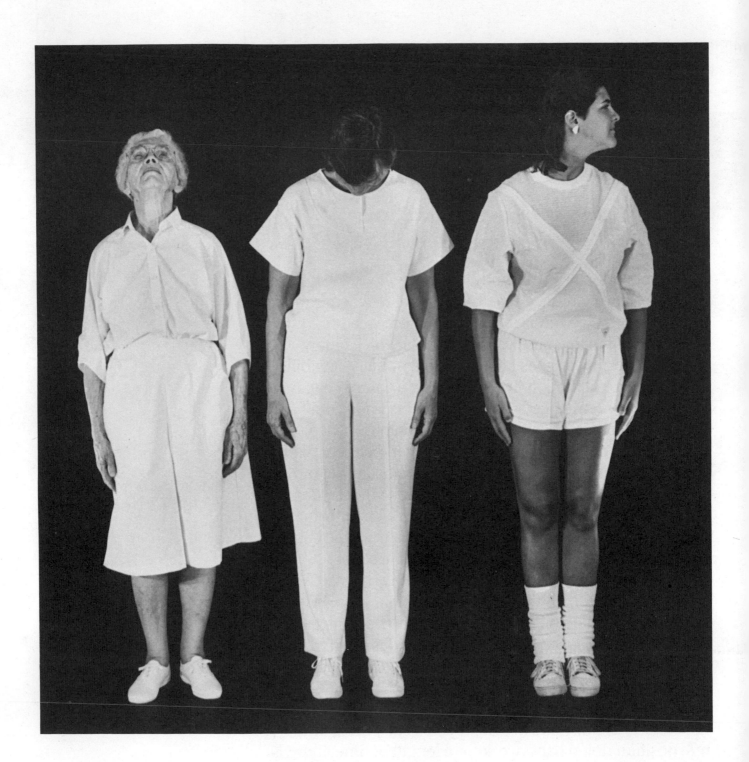

11. "HEAD-START"

A. Look up at the ceiling and let your head fall back as far as possible and hold it in that position for a bit.

B. Then slowly look down until your chin rests on your chest. Repeat the motions, up and down, up and down—slowly and gently.

C. Now turn your head from side to side, looking back and over your shoulder as far as possible. Do these motions slowly and steadily. Fast movements may cause a crink in your neck!

12. TURTLE SHRUG

A. Lift both shoulders up toward your ears, a deep turtle-neck shrug.

B. Now move shoulders back as far as possible, with chest out.

C. Now bring shoulders up again to the turtle-neck position.

D. Then drop shoulders to normal position. Repeat the motions—shoulders up, back, up and down. Relax arms and shoulders when in normal position.

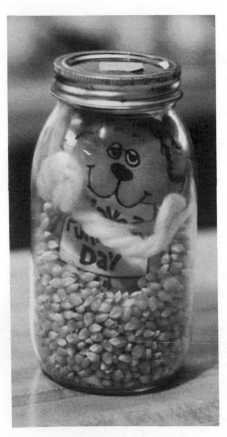

Grandma and I started an unusual tradition with a funny-looking little hot pink stuffed cat. It started because she told me about an ugly pincushion she and her sister Ida used to hide in each other's things. Since her sister's family lived abroad, the pincushion had crossed the ocean in various suitcases and barrels several times. It had also been baked in pies, cakes, and casseroles. Once it had been canned with some peaches. They were always coming up with creative ways to send it back to each other.

I thought this was too wonderful a tradition to discontinue, so I started a new one. I couldn't find an appropriate pincushion, so I bought an ugly stuffed cat instead. I hid it in her oatmeal box the first time and left a note with instructions about our tradition. A few days later I discovered the cat hanging in the shower room of my dorm at the college. Grandma had given it to my roommate to place there. Since then I have found it in my suitcase, under my bed, and wrapped for Christmas or my birthday. I never know where it will show up next. When Grandma has it, she says she sets it on her dresser with the family photographs.—Beth.

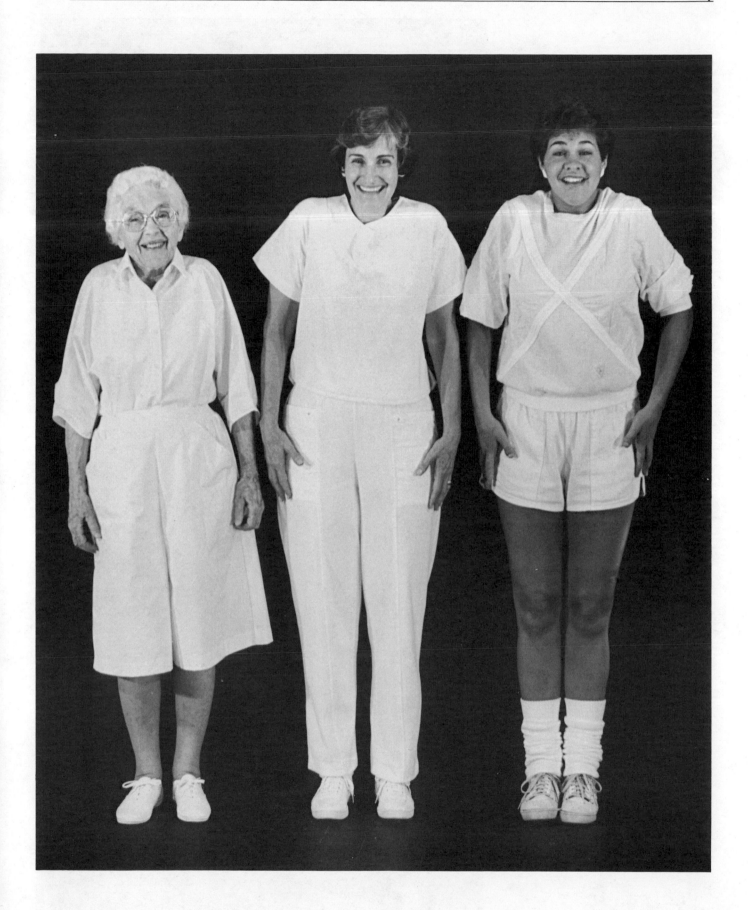

13. TILT AND STRETCH

A. Clasp your hands behind your back in a comfortable position.

B. Extend arms behind you and stretch them as far as possible, and at the same time

C. Tilt your head back as far as you can.

D. Bring your clasped hands to the middle of your back in a more relaxed position and drop your chin on your chest. Relax as much as possible and then repeat the sequence.

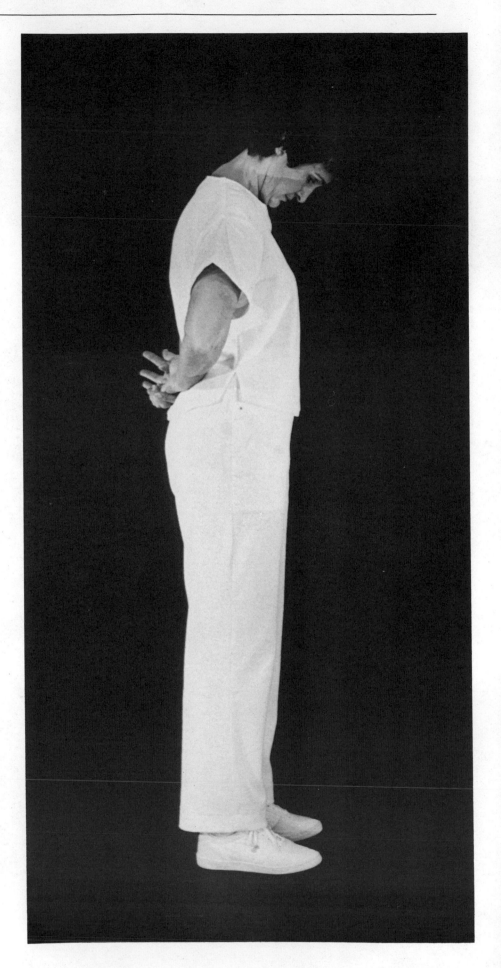

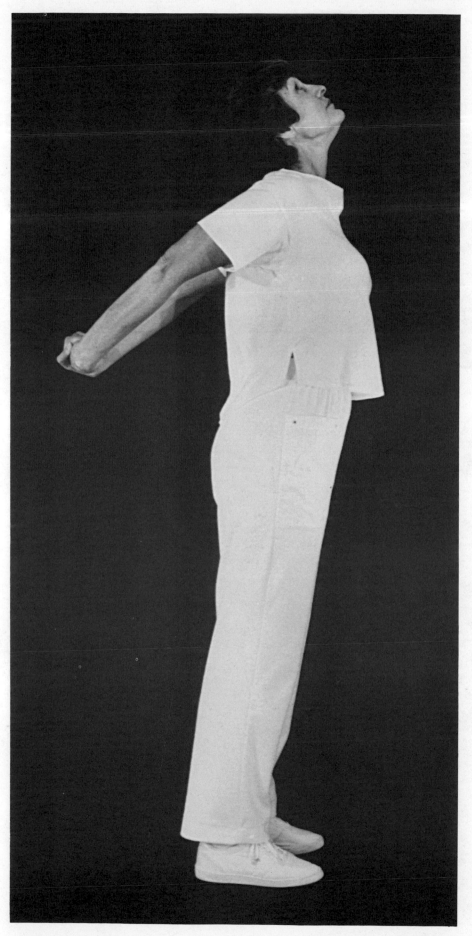

Northern Indiana usually receives a lot of snow during the winter. This was especially true one winter when I was in college there.

Grandma would often stand at her window, peering out at the world as it became blanketed in white. She had a gold four-door Plymouth Valiant which she parked within view of her window, and she would watch as it disappeared beneath a thick layer of snow.

My brother, Phil, was visiting her once when her car was covered with about six inches of snow. As she looked out at it, she said to him, "You know, my car looks like a cocoon. I keep hoping when the snow melts my Plymouth will have turned into a Buick."—Beth

14. TWISTERS

A. Raise your arms and extend them straight out at your sides at shoulder height. Have your feet apart a bit and bend your knees slightly.

B. Now twist from side to side slowly at the waist, swing-

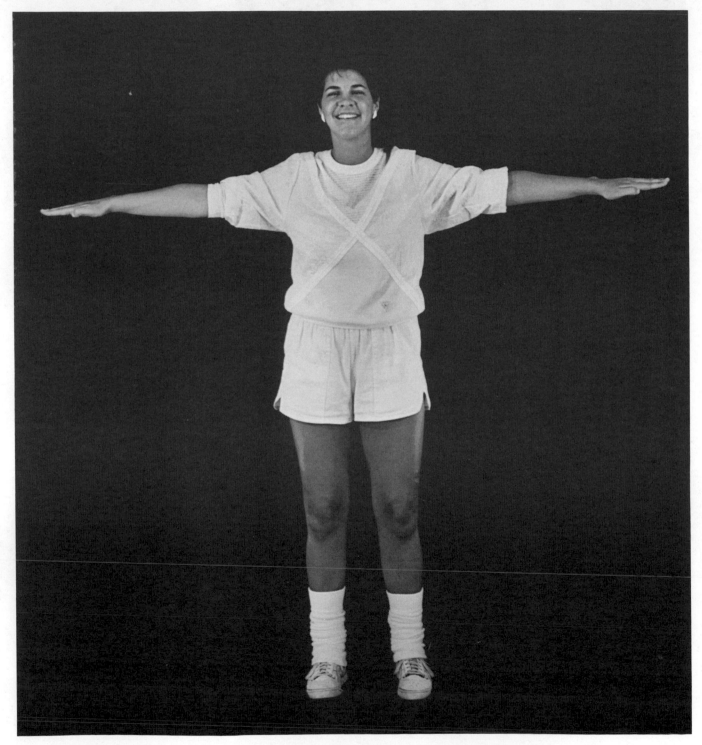

ing your arms. Try not to move your feet.
C. Don't hold your breath while you are twisting! Breathe in rhythm with your movements.
D. Increase speed and number as you are able.

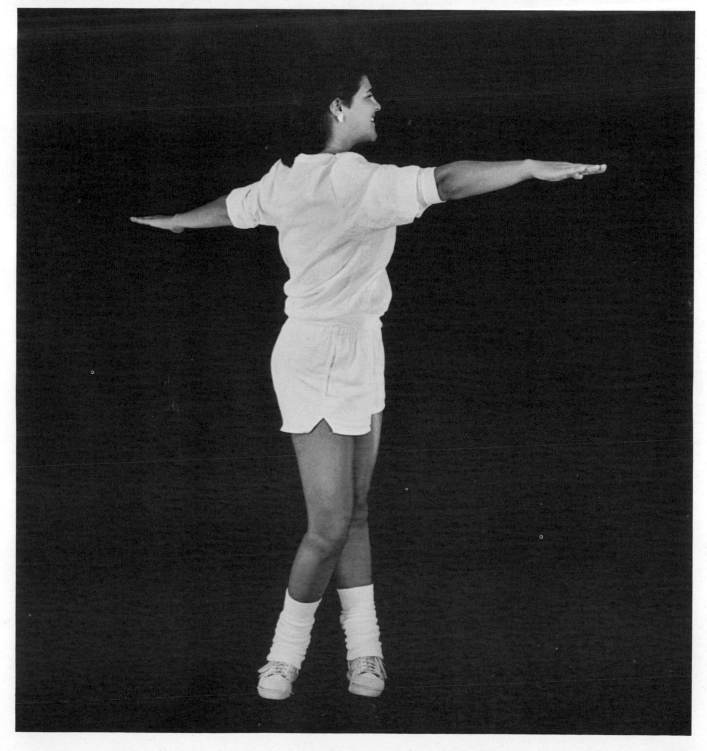

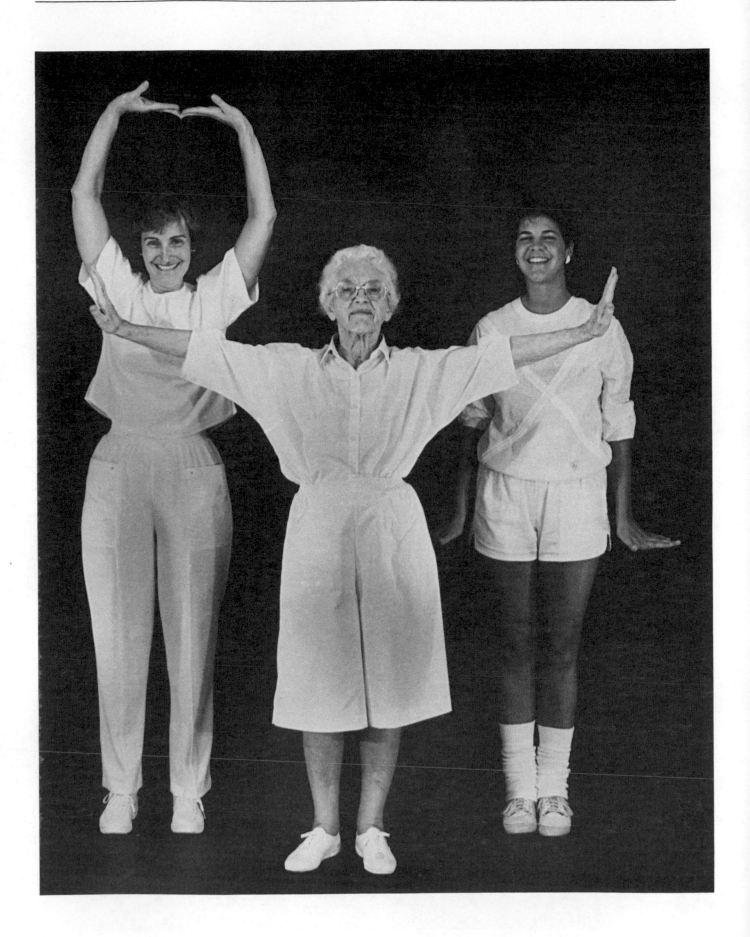

This exercise is designed to increase the flexibility of your shoulders and to enhance the tone of your arm muscles. As you go through these motions, exert some extra pull or tension so that you feel the tug in your upper arms and forearms. Repeat these motions as often as you can.

15. "PALM SPRINGS"

A. Put your hands above your head. Position hands, palms up, as though you were pushing up against the ceiling.

B. Now extend arms to the sides at shoulder level, with your hands still up and palms out.

C. Then bring arms down to your sides again, hands still up, palms toward the floor. Count—one, two, three— as you repeat the motions.

The next three exercises are to help keep your legs, hips and feet flexible and you will feel your thigh and back muscles working as well. You will need a chair for several of these.

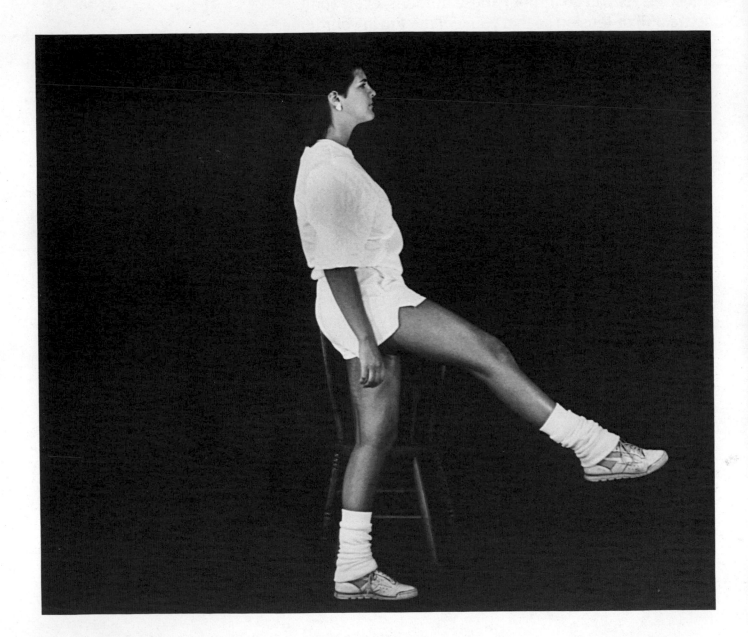

16. "CHAIR-DO"

A. Stand to the side of a chair, holding onto the back of it with your left hand.

B. Swing your right leg forward and up with your knee slightly bent.

C. Now swing your right leg all the way back and up.

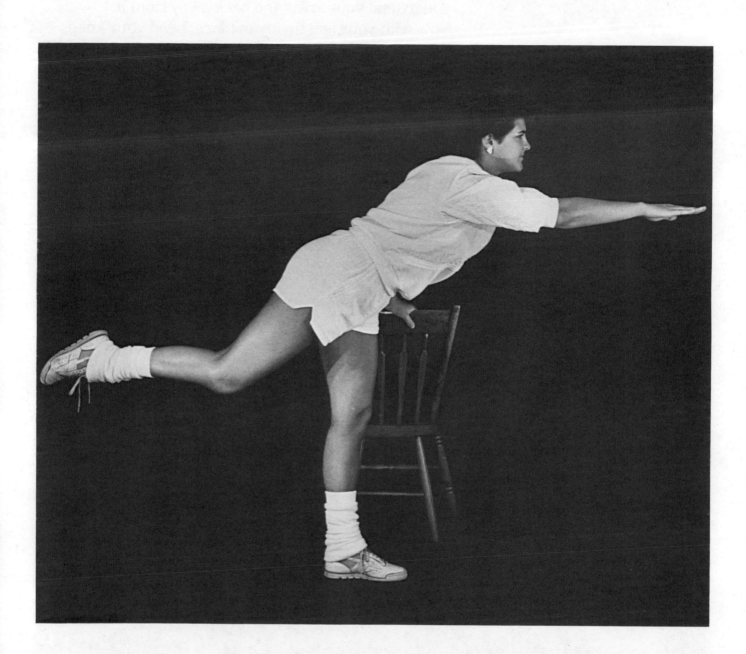

D. Go to the other side of the chair and hold onto the
    back of it with your right hand, and swing your left leg
    forward and up and then back and up. Increase and
    exaggerate the motions as you are able, moving your
    entire body with the motion.

17. "CHAIR-A-TEE"

A. Stand behind the chair and hold onto the back of it with both hands. Continue to hold onto the chair as you extend your arms and back away from it.

B. Now with your feet firmly in place, bend your knees slightly, and then bend over, putting your head between your arms.

C. It gets a bit more difficult! While holding onto the chair with your right hand, lean over to the left and touch your left hand to the floor. Then return both hands to the chair back.

D. Repeat those motions, leaning to the right side and touching the floor with your right hand and returning to the starting position.

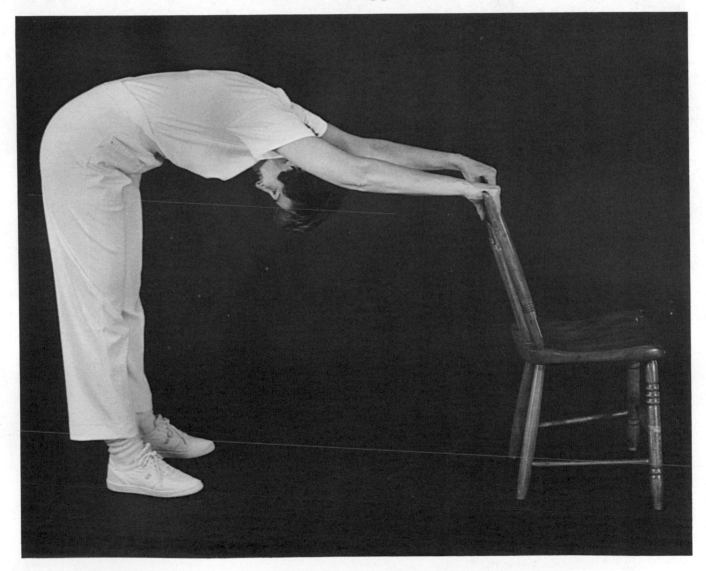

Our Pennsylvania Dutch Uncle Levi from Michigan was an Amish bishop. But when he visited at our home he easily laid aside the dignities of his office and became a great entertainer. We children were intrigued by his long white beard. One day my younger sister and I braided it into four braids and tied red ribbons on them. Suddenly we noticed a group of visitors coming toward the house. We were in a panic! The visitors were ushered into another room, while the braids were undone, the beard brushed out, and Uncle Levi put on his proper expression and went out to greet the guests.—Grandma

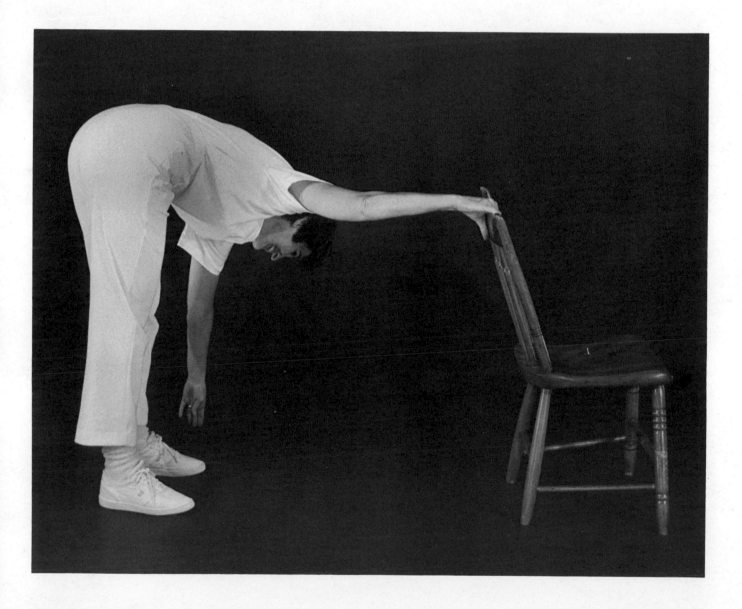

18. "CHAIR-EE-O"

A. You may hold onto the chair with one or both hands for this one.

B. Lift your right leg out in front of you and rotate your foot as though you are making a circle with your toe.

C. Repeat this same motion with your left leg and foot. Make at least 10 circles.

"Wear a smile and have friends. Wear a scowl and have wrinkles."

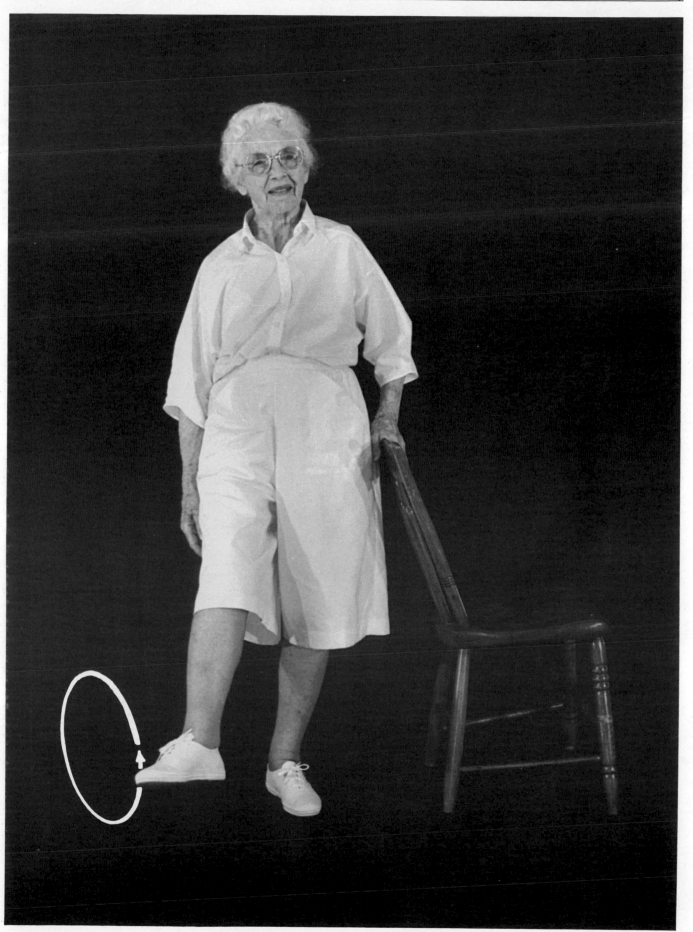

Since the shoulder is a ball and socket joint, this exercise will help maintain shoulder mobility as well as strengthen your upper arms. It may also tighten up some of that flab!

19. "ARMS REDUCTION"

A. Extend your arms straight out at your sides, at shoulder level.

B. Rotate your arms from the shoulder, clock-wise and then counter-clockwise. Make at least 10 good-sized circles with each arm.

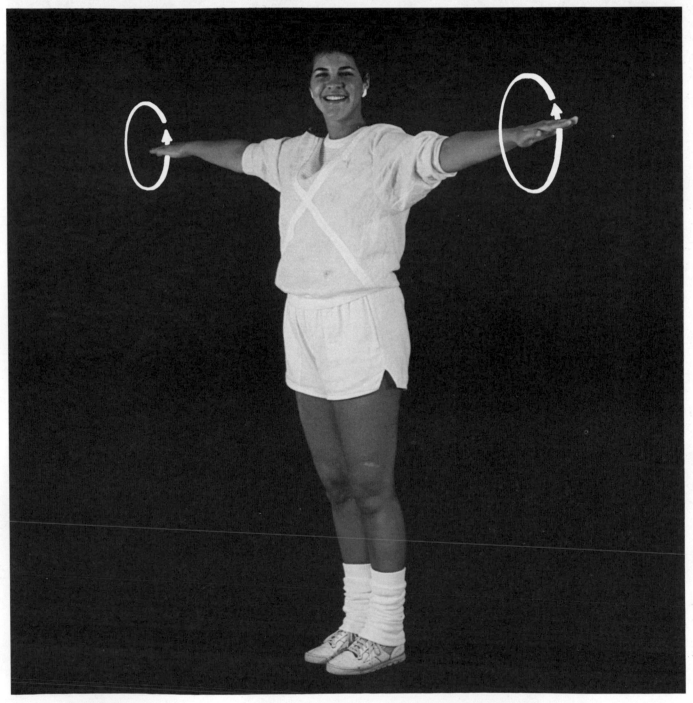

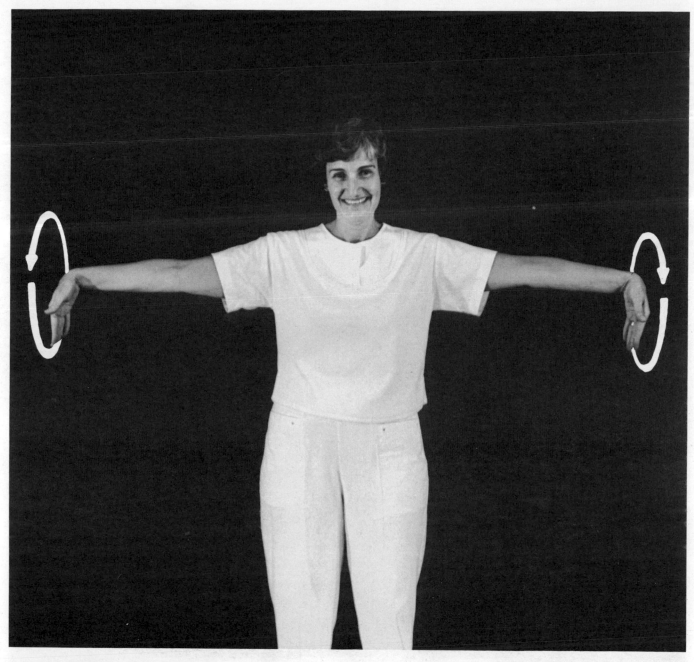

20. "WRIST WATCH"

A. Extend your arms straight out at your sides, again at shoulder level.

B. Rotate your wrists to make circles, about 10 times each.

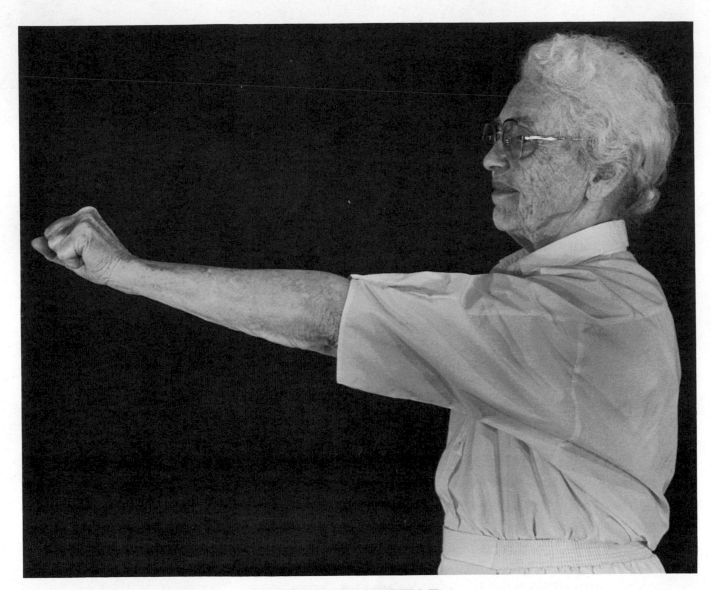

21. FINGER SPREAD

A. Extend your arms straight in front of you.
B. Now make a tight fist and hold it a few seconds.
C. Release the tension and spread your fingers, 10 times each.

There are so many daily activities and tasks of living that require your wrists and fingers to be flexible and agile. When you have finished these, try letting your arms and hands hang loosely at your sides, and then shake your hands vigorously and then your entire arm. This can relax you after exercising and tensing these muscles.

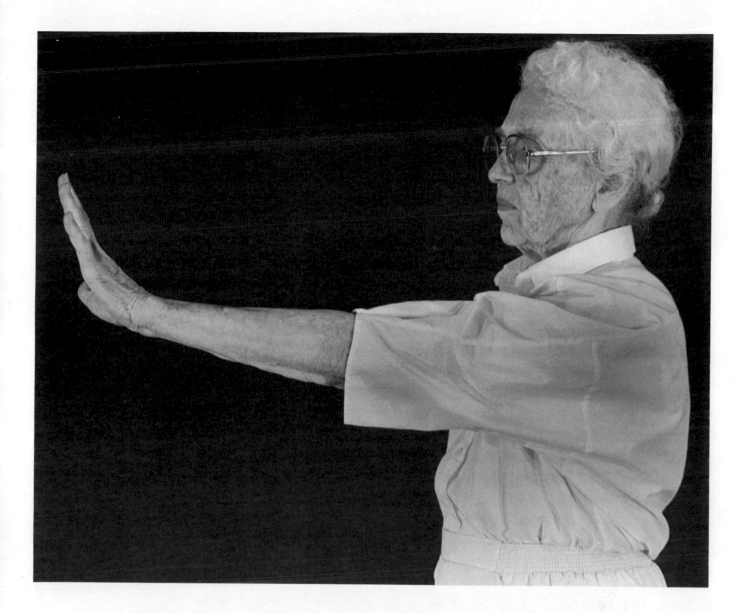

The next two exercises are good for increasing circulation in your legs. These are especially good if you spend a lot of time sitting during the day. When you think about it, just stretch your legs out and do these for a few minutes. It will relax some tension and keep the blood from pooling in your lower legs. Can you feel your abdominal muscles working, too?

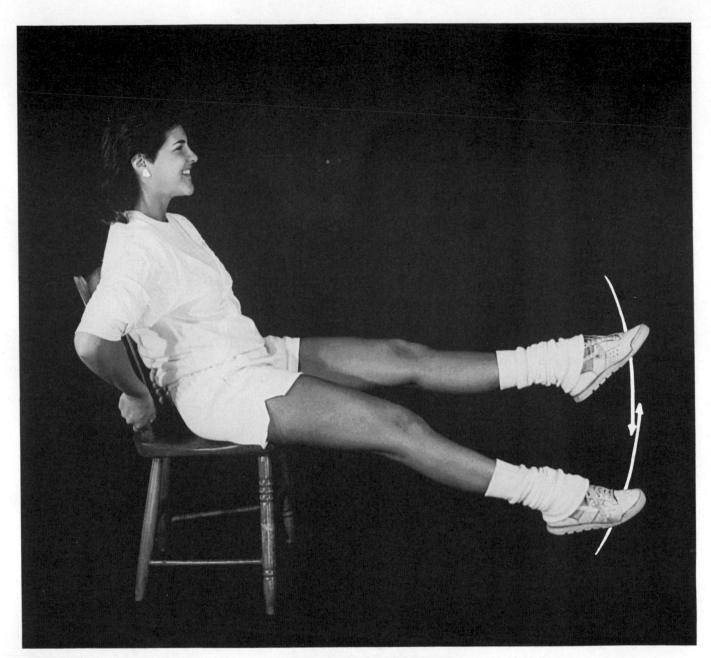

22. "PEDAL PUSHERS"

A. Sit at the front edge of a sturdy chair.
B. Extend your legs and keep them up off the floor eight or 10 inches. Point your toes.
C. Now do a scissors kick or a bicycle motion.

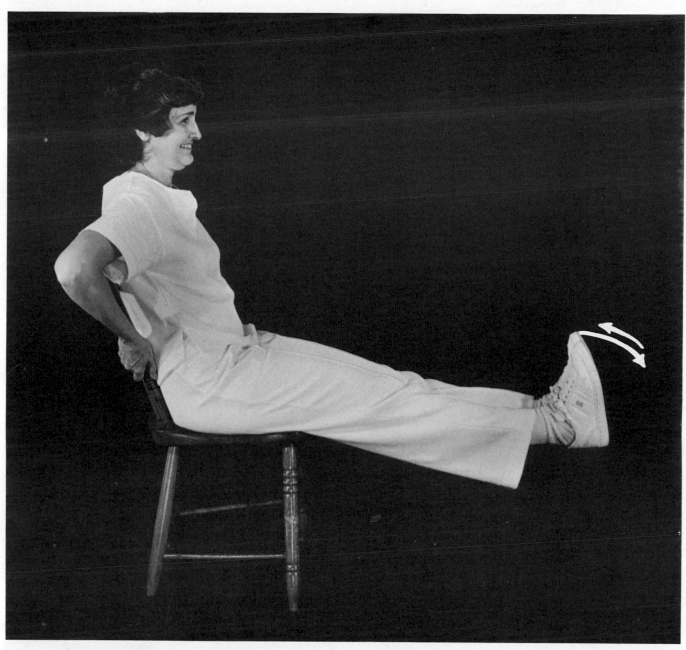

23. "TOE-STIR"

A. Sit up straight in your chair and extend your legs in front of you. Try to keep your legs together and point your toes.

B. Bring your toes up toward your knees and down again to the pointed position.

Exercises 24 and 25 will help you use many of the muscles in your legs, back and arms. You will soon feel which muscles feel tight and what you will need to work on to have more mobility and a wider range of motion. If you can't reach all the way at first, go as far as you can each time and increase it a bit each day.

24. "NONA'S KNEE-NOSE"

A. Sit on the edge of your chair and bring one knee at a time up to touch your nose. Do this slowly! Right knee—left knee—right knee—left knee.

B. Keep your back as straight as possible. You will probably feel a need to bend down toward your knee.

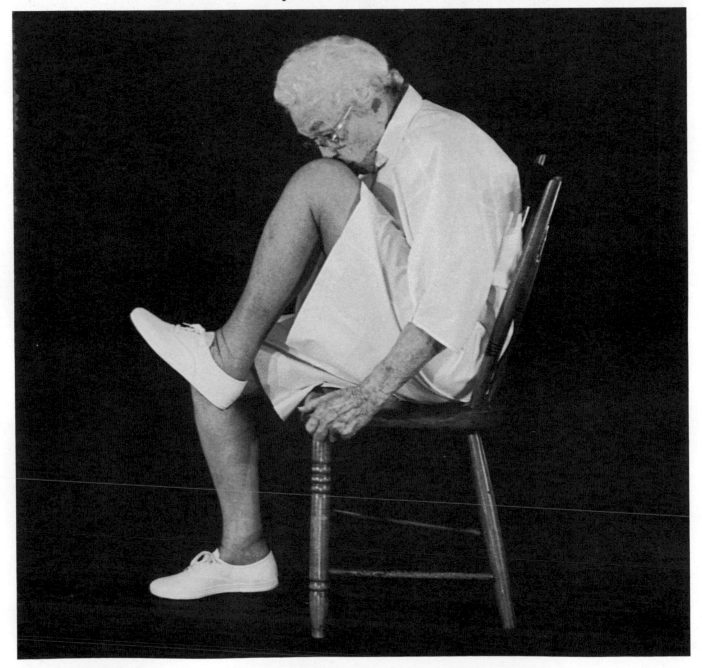

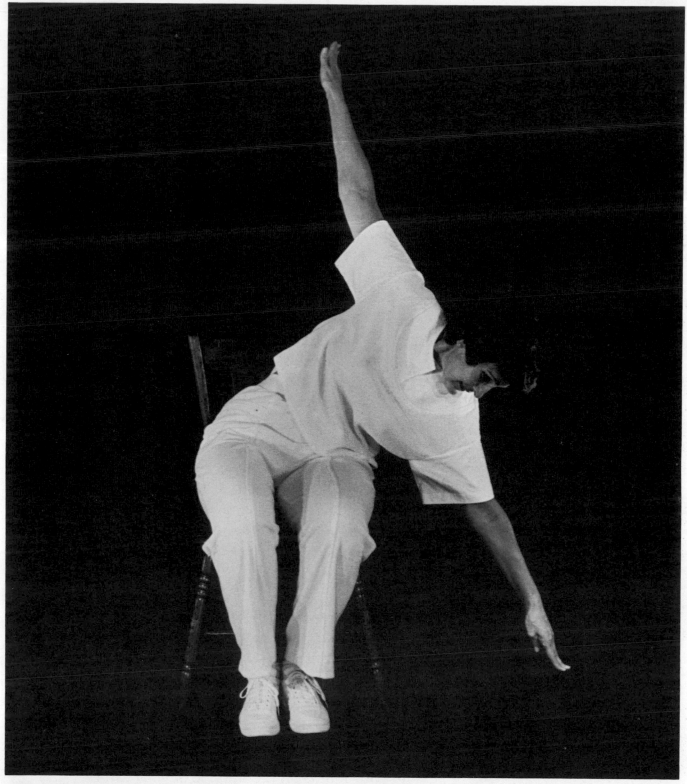

25. "LEAN-TO"

A. Sit up straight and extend your arms to shoulder level.
B. Now lean to the left side until you can touch the floor
    with your left hand. Try to keep your knees together.
C. Then reverse the motion and touch the floor with your
    right hand.

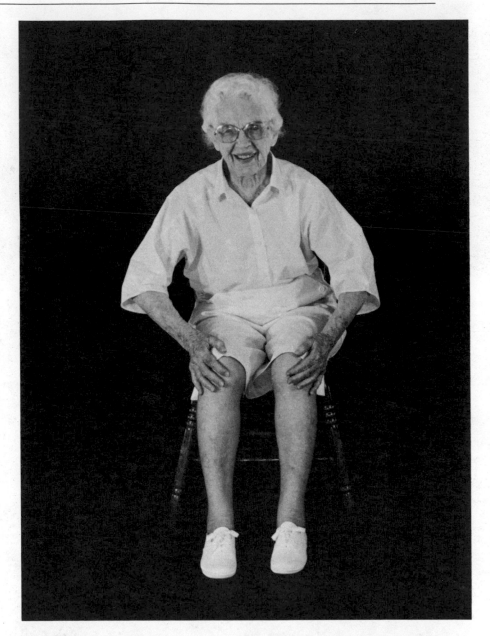

The next exercise is what is called an isotonic exercise. That means that a muscle group is forced against some resistance. These do not do much for circulation but are good to increase muscle strength.

26. "KNEES-SQUEEZE"

A. Place your feet firmly and comfortably on the floor, and your hands on the *outside* of your knees.

B. Try to push your knees apart, but resist that motion with your hands.

C. Now place hands on the *inside* of your knees and try to push your knees *together*. Resist this motion with your hands. Push hard enough so that you can feel the muscles in your arms, as well as your legs, really working.

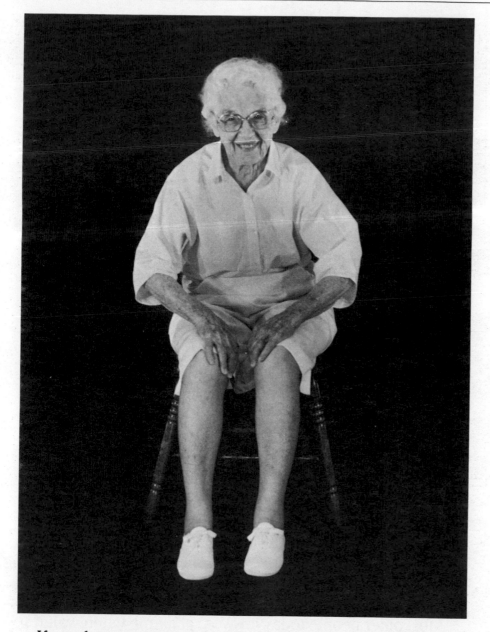

If you have progressed to the point where you are able to do a series of active exercises for 20 minutes or more without a break, you will want to cool down or unwind when you are finished. This can be done in the same way you warmed up. Walk around as you move your shoulders up and down. Put your hands on your hips and turn from side to side a few times. Take some deep breaths, let your shoulders drop forward and your arms dangle loosely. Dr. Kantner suggests a cool-down period of at least 10% of the time you spent in vigorous exercise. □

7

Walking Your Own Mile

Walking has been practiced for centuries by many poets, philosophers and religious folks who realized its benefits. They talked about it in terms of walking to cleanse the spirit, to lift the soul, to meditate and to pray. Ralph Waldo Emerson wrote, " . . . Few men know how to take a good walk. The qualifications are endurance, plain clothes, old shoes, an eye for Nature, good humor, vast curiosity, good speech and good silence." Plato said that walking is so relaxing "it could almost relieve a guilty conscience."

There are a lot of things to remind us of what we call, with some nostalgia, the "good old days"—old furniture, wood-burning stoves, lamps, butter churns, baskets, antique dishes, you name it. However, the old-fashioned idea that walking is better than riding doesn't seem to elicit the same nostalgia.

Walking Is a Way of Life

Most older people today grew up at a time when walking was not for exercise—it was a necessity. Stories about how far grandparents walked to school and work are repeated, usually to admonish someone younger when they complain about having to walk to school.

Few of us can remember when we first started walking, but those first baby steps are universally encouraged and applauded. Calls to grandparents, picture-taking and even bronzing baby shoes indicate the importance of walking. "Does he walk yet?" is asked almost as often as the baby's name and age. Many children can walk by age one but as they grow up into adolescents, they are still working at gaining control over their bodies for walking. Sometimes it seems as children grow taller and more gangly, they must

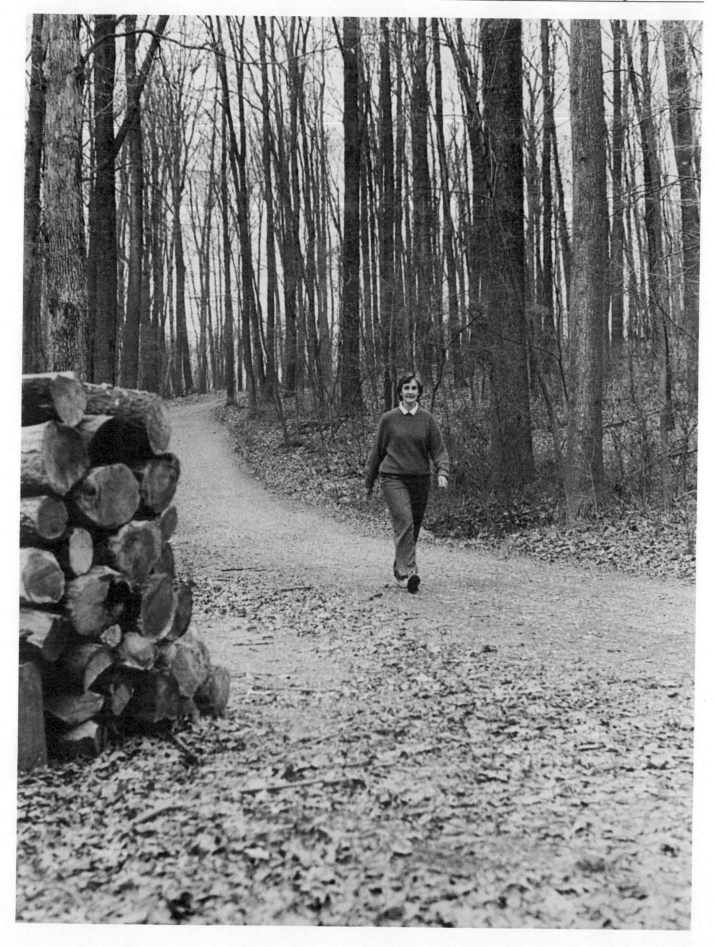

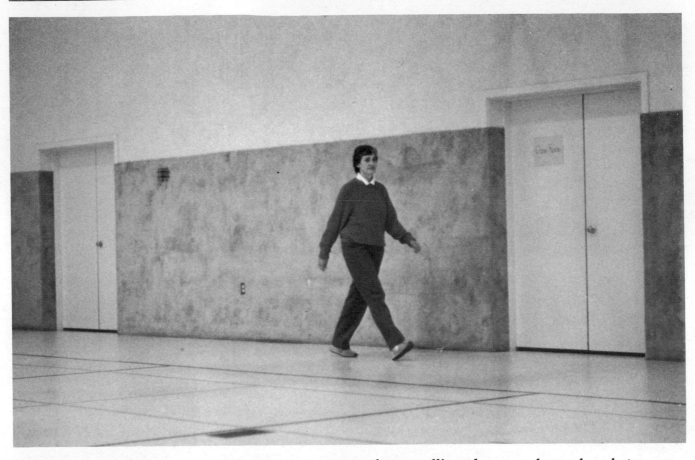

learn a new way of controlling those awkward and strange things under them called legs and feet!

Each person walks differently, with a style as unique as individual signatures.[4] We can recognize people from a distance by the way they walk. Posture, gait, the way the head is held, stride and balance, all say something about that individual. Remember trying to imitate someone's walk either for fun or because you admired them?

Regardless of unique styles or gaits, walking is a series of movements that propel us forward, body passing over each supporting leg as the other swings forward for the next support phase. In contrast to running or jumping, during walking, one foot is always on the ground.

As we walk our bodies move in several directions. There is movement up and down, but there is also a slight movement from side to side, and of course forward and backward. All this is done in a connected and systematic way. Your body may appear to be in continuous forward motion, but it is actually slowing down and speeding up as each step is taken. With all the shifting and rotating from head to toe, nearly all parts of the body are in motion at some time when we are walking. It is truly amazing that these many separate movements are coordinated and rhythmic!

As we have said before, exercises that assist you to proper conditioning are those that are continuous, rhythmic, and get your muscles to pump repeatedly. Walking can be one of these. Your blood pressure can be lowered, your resting heart rate decreased and your muscles, including your heart muscle, can become stronger and more efficient.

Let's talk about these kind of exercises in terms of aerobic exercises.

The word aerobic means air, but actually refers more to the oxygen in the air. Since your muscles need oxygen to function, their need for oxygen is increased, often quite dramatically, when you are giving them a workout. It follows then, that as you exercise more vigorously, you need more oxygen and your heart rate goes up. Aerobic exercises will make the muscles work hard enough to need more oxygen, but not so hard as to exceed the heart's ability to deliver it.

An Ideal Aerobic Exercise

Aerobic exercises are defined as those steady exercises that call for an uninterrupted output from your muscles over a period of time, at least 12 to 20 minutes. This kind of exercise maximizes the amount of oxygen your body can process or deliver throughout your body in a given time. Jogging, running, swimming or walking are examples of this kind of exercise that improves the health of your heart, lungs and vascular system. The result is a conditioning or training effect which short bursts of exercise do not produce.

To exercise in a most efficient way, you should be aware of what is happening to your heart rate as you walk or exercise. This is because your aerobic capacity, or the body's ability to pick up oxygen and send it throughout your body, is an important way of measuring the effectiveness of your activity. Your aerobic capacity is improved when your heart begins to beat faster, and your need for oxygen is increased. Your blood vessels expand to carry these larger amounts of oxygen-rich blood to the brain and torso, which is what you want to happen.

As a child I remember my father telling me about a leg injury he had when he was young. As a result he walked with a particular stride, one long step—one shorter step. I could feel the rhythm and imitated it as I held his hand when we walked.

We were on a party phone line then and "central" would ring us when we had a call; one long ring—one shorter ring, one long ring—one shorter ring. I used to think she did that because she knew how my dad walked.
—Naomi

As you walk, your muscles, especially in your arms and legs, are getting a work-out. Unused blood vessels begin to open, which allows a good pick-up of oxygen. Cardiologists sometimes refer to the leg motion of walking as a "second heart."[5] This is because when you walk, your thighs and calf muscles help to squeeze blood back toward the heart from the feet and legs where blood tends to pool.

Aerobic walking then, is walking with speed and effort, any style, for at least 20 minutes. This can train your heart and lungs. Your breathing capacity is also increased because of the expansion of the chest and lungs.

There are other benefits from walking. You are working at balance and coordination as well as poise and posture. Some walking enthusiasts insist that walking also improves sexual performance because physical stamina is increased and the mental stimulation keeps you in better touch with the senses. There are health and fitness programs designed to specifically improve sexual intimacy between marriage partners.

Walking has less potential for injuries and is a most natural function for these bodies of ours. There is none of that pounding trauma to knees and joints that can come from jogging or running. It can relieve stress, improve problem-solving ability, help relieve depression, and give you a sense of self-control. It allows you to eat well without gaining weight and stimulates elimination as well.

Of course, other exercises can do all those things, too, but the only exercises that can benefit you are the ones you *do*. Walking is one that most people *can* do! The benefit of walking, or any exercise, can be measured by the duration, intensity, and frequency of that exercise, as well as which muscle groups are used.

When Is Walking Exercise?

"Life is a continual battle between keeping your spirits up and your weight down."

So how can you measure when walking is really an exercise? Remember that you are not like anyone else. Don't compare yourself with others. There are, however, three "tests" you can take to see if the intensity and duration of your walking is truly beneficial to you:

1. Pain Test: You should not experience pain as you walk. If you do, your body is trying to tell you something, so listen. Do your shoes fit well? Maybe you need to slow

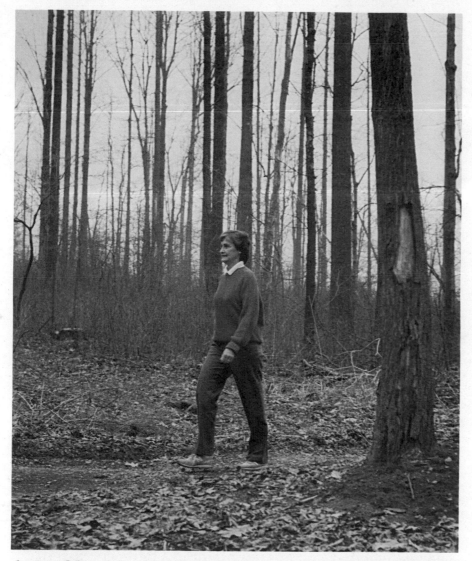

Both our sons began walking before they were a year old, but they were reluctant to let go of our fingers as we steered them along and helped with their balance. We put round clothespins in their hands which they clasped eagerly, and went on their way, practicing their walking skills, hanging onto two clothespins.—Naomi

down. Of course, if pain continues, see your physician.

2. Talk Test: Even though you may walk by yourself, you should have enough breath and energy to talk with someone. If you don't feel as though you are able to talk, you are likely walking too fast for your age and condition. This is especially important if you are just beginning to walk for exercise.

3. Tired Test: If you tend to feel quite tired for an hour or more after your walk, your walk was likely too strenuous.

Dr. Kenneth Cooper, in his book *The Aerobics Way,* suggests a rough rule of thumb to find out how fast you are walking. Determine the number of steps you take per minute. If you are walking at 90 steps per minute, you should be able to cover a mile in about 20 minutes. A 15-minute mile is 120 steps per minute and that is travelling at a good clip. [6]

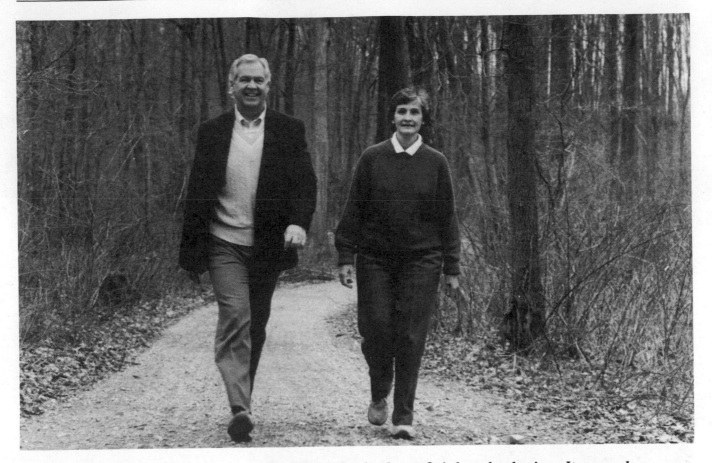

Strolling can be beneficial and relaxing. It may also improve your circulation but will not train your heart to perform better.

There is another way to know when walking is an exercise which benefits you. You can use your heart rate to measure whether you are maintaining a fairly consistent level of effort. And as you may guess, there are a number of ways to figure what is called a Target Heart Rate Range or Zone. You need to be able to take your pulse which tells how fast your heart is beating.

You will need a watch with a second hand to count your pulse rate. You can usually feel your pulse just inside your wrist, below your thumb, by placing two or three fingers lightly on this area. This is over the radial artery. Don't use your thumb to count your pulse because the thumb has a pulse of its own and can be confused with the radial pulse you are trying to count. Count the beats for 15 seconds and multiply by four.

This should be done when you are at rest. Your goal will be to increase this heart rate as you walk and exercise. An increase will mean that you are benefiting from the exercise. Generally speaking, the better shape you are in, the slower your heart at rest will be. A slower pulse at rest means that your heart is accomplishing its task with less beats.

To take your pulse when you are exercising or walking, simply count the beats for six seconds and then multiply by 10. This will be the number of beats per minute. It may be easier to take your pulse by feeling your throat just below your ear. Use your fingertips and slide them down from your ear, just under your jaw bone (or to the side of your voice box) until you can feel your pulse. Don't press too hard.

To find your Target Heart Rate Range:
    Subtract your age from 220
        Multiply by .70
        Multiply by .80

Example: If you are 70 years old; take 220 minus 70 years which equals 150. Then take 150 times .70 which equals 105. And 150 times .80 equals 120. According to this scale your Target Heart Rate Range would be 105 to 120 beats per minute. This means that when you exercise and your heart beats between 105 and 120 beats per minute, you are exercising within a safe and efficient range.

Easy Does It

Even though we have talked about the importance of training your heart and the benefits of aerobic exercises, we want to emphasize again that, especially for older people, it is important to plan a program of exercise with your physician's approval. The intensity, duration, frequency, and kinds of exercises which will be helpful should be planned and supervised for your particular needs and condition (see Chapter 2). If your personal physician does not seem particularly interested in assisting you, ask for referral to a physician who could help you.

Start slowly if you have not been doing any kind of exercise or much walking. Some physicians feel you should spend at least one month getting yourself in condition for every year you have been sedentary. For example, if you are just beginning, walk only 10 minutes a day three or four times a week. See how you feel, listen to your body and increase or decrease the time and frequency until you are ready to move to 12 or 15 minutes three or four times

It is curious what I remember about our wedding day. When John and I stood before my preacher father who married us, my mind wandered back to the many times when in his gentle way he had supported and encouraged me. But the thing I remember most clearly as he spoke to us was looking at his eyes and noticing the white paint speckles on his glasses. He had helped us paint the home into which we would move. At that moment I loved my father dearly.—Naomi

a week.

Don't think too much about the speed you walk at first; walk the amount of time you have set. Take your pulse and if it is below the Target Heart Range that you calculated, then you are pacing yourself about right for a beginner. As you progress, you can get your heart rate up within the Target Heart Range. If you are interested, then, in really improving your fitness level, you should walk at your Target Heart Range for at least 20 minutes three or four times a week.

Your breathing should be slow and rhythmic if you are walking slowly. Inhale for the first step and exhale for the next step. If you are walking faster, inhale during two steps and exhale during two steps. Whatever you choose, your breathing should be rhythmic and synchronized with your leg and arm movements. Be aware of breathing and count if that helps.

When you walk, stand up straight and keep your eyes ahead if possible (don't stumble on anything!). Shoulders should be relaxed and your back should not be hunched up. When you walk faster, you tend to lean forward and your shoulders may hunch up which can cause some discomfort. Have a friend watch you as you walk and see what they say about your walking posture. Arms can swing loosely at your sides or be bent at the elbow if you are walking rapidly. Try to be aware of extra movements up and down or from side to side that may take extra energy and distract from a smooth, comfortable style.

Comfortable and Safe

"It is not the load that gets you down, it's the way you carry it."

Although Emerson thought an old pair of shoes was good enough, we insist that, old or not, they are good, sturdy, supportive shoes. The shoes should be flexible, have plenty of toe room with a cushioned sole and support of the heel and arch. The material they are made of should "breathe" and not be heavy.

Running shoes generally meet these requirements. For some persons however, running shoes may have heels too low for comfort. Remember that your feet hit the ground about 400 times a mile! Be kind to them.

Emerson did have a point when he talked about *old* shoes. Break in new shoes before you try to walk too far.

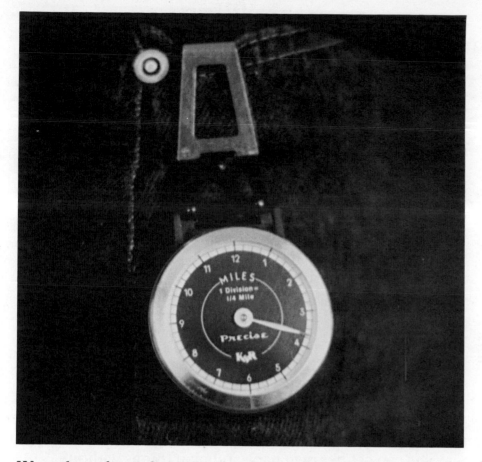

Wear them for a short time each day before you set out on a longer walk. Wear heavy socks to help prevent blisters.

You may occasionally experience muscle soreness even though you walk regularly. Keep walking, but cut down a bit on speed and distance until you feel ready to go again. If you experience pain in the calf of your leg, you may do better with a little higher heel.

To massage your aching feet, squeeze each foot with both hands. Muscle cramps can occur but are less likely if you do some warm-ups and stop before you are really fatigued.

It is also advisable to wait for an hour or more after a meal to do any kind of exercises or speedy walking. If you get a stitch in your side, bend forward and inhale deeply and push your abdomen in and out. As we have said many times before, listen to your body and if pain or discomfort persists, see your physician before you continue exercising or walking for exercise.

Lightweight, loose-fitting, comfortable clothes are best to wear. Consider also that clothes which are bright can be seen more easily by motorists than darker ones. Dress warmly (but not too warmly!) in cold weather and wear cotton clothes in warm weather. If it is very cold or very hot weather, consider exercising indoors. Drink enough water to stay hydrated, especially if you perspire a lot.

Walk safely, too! If you are walking on a road, face the oncoming traffic. If it is getting dark, wear a belt or strap made of reflective material. It is best to walk on a familiar route and to know where you are going.

In very cold or inclement weather, Grandma walks up and down and all around the halls in the retirement center where she lives. Since she has a pedometer, she ticks off the miles in style! You could simply walk in place, too, although this is not as interesting. Music that suits the style and speed of your walk may add to the ease with which you can walk in place, and make it more interesting at the same time.

Give your mother or grandmother a
pedometer for Christmas!

You may like to walk with someone, not only to keep you company, but to help you with the discipline of actually getting out and walking. Grandma likes to walk alone. That way she can set her own pace and plan things without being interrupted! She thinks about how she will sew a new blouse or get ready for a talk she will be giving or work on how she will teach her Sunday school class.

Let your walking be a time to be stimulated by sounds and sights around you. Grandma repeats poetry she has learned over the years. You can become your own best company.

Walk your own mile. Set your own long-range goals such as walking one-half to one or two miles a day. Expect to progress slowly and gradually over a period of six months or a year, especially if you are a beginner. ☐

"Things are not so much impossible as they are untried."

Fit, Fat, Philosophy, and Bran

8

We can hardly talk about exercise, energy output, and the benefits of activity without also taking a look at what we eat and the effect that has on our general health. So much has been written about diets, how to lose weight, what is good for you and what is not, it is indeed hard to know what to believe. There are a few ideas that are important and can be used as guidelines to good nutrition.

"Progress" in Consumption?

The average American diet can be hazardous to your health. Consider what has been called "progress" in the consumption of food. Since the beginning of the 19th century, the more efficient milling process for flour has actually caused flour to have a deficiency of vitamin B. Preservatives, pre-packaged, processed foods, soft drinks, and salty and sweetened snack foods all add to our dilemma. Of course, there were hazards related to diets of generations ago, but we do have a new set of opportunities and responsibilities as we make choices about what we eat.

There is also a new way or style of eating that can be reason for concern. Someone has said the "death of the family table" is as much responsible for our poor eating habits as anything. Families no longer sit down together to eat their meals. Each member has a schedule to meet, with sports, job, church, and various community activities placing demands upon them. It is simply hard to find a time when everyone is at home at the same time. Fast food restaurants and convenience foods, plus microwave ovens, have also helped change family eating habits.

As family members get older and children move away, many of us find ourselves cooking for only one or two people. It becomes difficult to plan meals and is sometimes easier not to cook at all. While it is true that we need less calories as we get older, it does not change our need for a balance of foods to maintain good nutrition.

On the other hand, some persons do actually overeat. There are extraordinarily high numbers of obese people in North America. This is primarily due to general physical inactivity along with a high calorie intake. We eat more than our bodies need.

Deficiencies in vitamins and minerals from poor or unbalanced diets can cause a whole list of problems. Our initial response may be to go out and buy all kinds of food supplements and vitamins to fill this need. This is appealing to older people as well as to those living on the run since we seem to have the notion that we can take a pill to make us healthy, or that someone has indeed found a great new cure for whatever ails us. To add to our confusion, the media floods us with information about what supplements or certain foods will or won't do, what is harmful and what is healthy.

Books on good nutrition abound (there are a number listed in the annotated bibliography). But let us also suggest a few important things that have to do with the philosophy of food and eating, as well as some more concrete suggestions about a balanced diet.

Nutrition for a Healthy Life

The philosophy of this book is that exercise can be simple, can be done by ordinary people without a lot of cost and equipment, and can help you toward a healthy life. This carries over into our beliefs about how and what we eat.

We as North Americans have, for the most part, lived at a time when food has been adequate if not abundant. Along with that, we spend a far lower percentage of our incomes for food than do most people in the world. We tend to eat too many calories, too much protein, too much sugar, too much salt, too much fat, and too many processed foods. We should eat to conserve resources in the world, and also to improve our own health.

We can:

1. Eat more whole grains, such as rice, wheat and oats. Include legumes such as dried beans and peas. Vegetables

Breakfast has always been important in our home. I grew up eating oatmeal, toast and fruit almost every morning. Grandma said she could tell which of her students had oatmeal for breakfast—they were the bright ones! It was most certainly a ploy to get us to eat oatmeal without complaining, but she did have a point!—Naomi

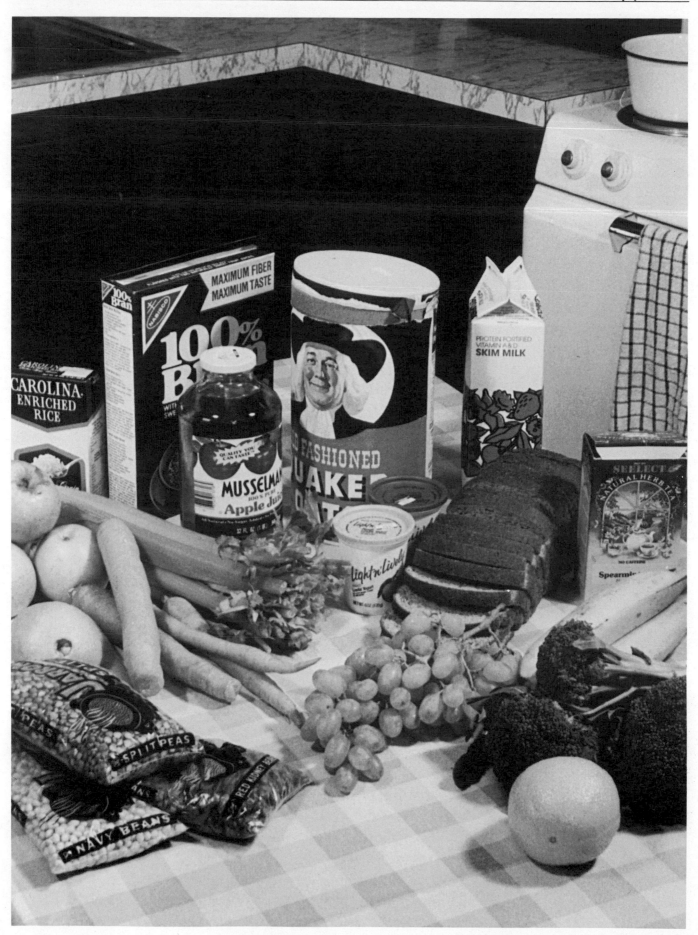

and fruits are always important and provide variety as well as necessary vitamins.

2. Use eggs, poultry, and meats in more limited amounts.

3. Avoid superpackaged foods and foods heavy in refined sugar or with a high sodium content. Avoid saturated fats and fried foods. Remember a variety of foods adds not only to the spice in your life but also to good nutrition.

If you are a little overweight, a lot overweight or obese, see your physician for a good, nutritious diet that will provide what you need to stay healthy and, at the same time, allow you to lose those pounds you don't need, and that may be, in fact, harmful.

Don't even *think* about going on a diet that suggests you eat only such things as grapefruit or protein as a way to magically lose weight. Any diet that recommends no carbohydrates, or all protein, or total elimination of certain foods may indeed lead to poor nutrition.

Use Your Common Sense

Use your good common sense. For example, if you know that your cholesterol count is high and you have been eating four eggs a day, you would be wise to cut down to only one or two a week. Yolks are the part of the egg that contains the cholesterol, so eat the whites if you like.

It's not all bad to treat yourself once a week to something you really like. That can satisfy your craving for a while and will allow you to stick to your diet better. The point is that a good way to lose weight is to decrease food intake and increase exercise in a way that allows your body to maintain proper balance.

Very simply, a good diet will include fruits, vegetables, protein, or combinations of plant proteins (rice and beans, for example), high fiber foods (oats, bran or whole wheat bread), and even a *few* of those sweet things you like.

Avoid fats and use low-fat milk and milk products. Bake, steam or broil your foods. Avoid refined sugar and excess salt. Drink plenty of fluids, other than coffee and tea. Water is best, but fruit juices and herbal teas without caffeine are also acceptable. With lots of fluids and a serving of bran, plus your exercises, you shouldn't have a problem with constipation. As you grow older, you may lose your desire

Grandma often prepares a "one pan" meal, especially at noon. She uses a little steam rack in a pan with enough water to reach the rack. Then she cuts up a potato and whatever other vegetable she wants, adds one-half a raw apple and an uncooked egg in the shell, and steams it till done to her taste. It doesn't take long and with a slice of whole-wheat bread and a glass of milk, it makes a delicious, simple and nutritious meal.—Naomi

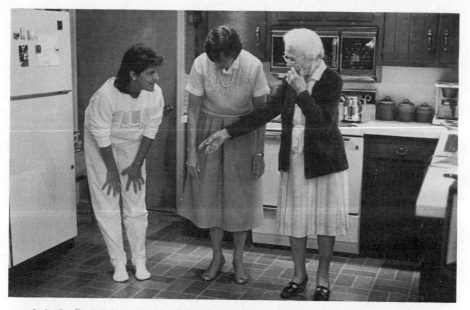

to drink fluids, but lack of fluids can be a problem.

It is a good idea to have one complete meal a day. It is easy just to snack on starchy foods that do not have much nutritional value.

Do you need extra vitamins and minerals? The best way to be sure you will get all the vitamins you need is to eat a wide variety of foods. There are those times when taking daily vitamins may be important. Current medical advice includes taking calcium tablets, especially for women who are approaching menopause or are postmenopausal. Ask your physician about this. Choose a physician who is truly interested in good nutrition, total fitness, education and prevention and not just in treating illness; one who will take time to talk about your nutritional needs.

Eating right is a part of total fitness. Eating right can also be eating simply. It is not just sprinkling bran or wheat germ over highly sugared cereal or ice cream and eating bean sprouts! It may mean making choices to change your basic philosophy about foods and their preparation.

We have changed our diets to choosing more simple foods, eating almost no red meat but some fish and poultry, and consuming very few fried foods, but lots of fresh fruits, vegetables and whole grain products. We made these choices not only for fitness and health, but because we want to be responsible consumers and aware of those around the world who may have limited food resources. Simple food cooked creatively can also be the best. ☐

Grandma's father told the children when they came to meals and protested something that was served, "You may say you don't like something or you don't care for that just now, but you must never say it isn't good. Your mother does not put anything on the table that is not good."—Beth

9 Putting It Together

Although this is the concluding chapter, it is, we hope, only the beginning. Regardless of what age or shape you are in, begin to think enough of yourself and your body to work toward fitness. You are the only one who can choose how to care for yourself, and whether you will actually become more active.

Design exercises which suit your individual needs. If you want to use a bit more energy with the ones we have suggested, hold a book or weights in your hands as you do them to make your muscles work a little harder.

Swimming is an almost perfect exercise since it puts nearly every major muscle to use and causes no stress points on the body because of the buoyancy of the water.

If you have special limitations such as arthritis or heart or back problems, you can still find tailor-made activities to enhance your well-being. Your mobility, flexibility, coordination, and balance can improve, as can the way you feel about yourself. Remember, you will need advice and consent from your physician regarding the kinds of activities that will benefit you.

Time and Times

In the book of Ecclesiastes in the Bible, the writer reflects about what life means and what good we can find in it. In the third chapter are these words:

For everything there is a season, and a time for every matter under heaven:

a time to be born, a time to die; . . .
a time to weep, and a time to laugh; . . .
a time to mourn and a time to dance; . . .

This book is also about time—and times. It is about reflecting and remembering, about laughing and crying, about serious and silly things. We believe that people can learn to live in a positive and productive way, as long as possible.

Naomi:

Grandma has made it so clear in the way she has lived that death is a part of life and not an end. She has shown us how to grow old. She believes that aging is the "master work of wisdom" and undeniably one of the most difficult chapters in the art of living.

I have often heard her say that nothing will happen to her that she and God cannot handle together. We as a family have experienced God's love in some dark and unhappy times, and in those times we have also remembered what we have learned and experienced during the many times of great joy.

Grandma has made and paid for all her funeral arrangements. These preparations were not because of a morbid or dreary preoccupation with death, but because it is part of the way she lives, optimistically and gratefully, knowing the time of her death, like her life, is in God's loving care.

While it is true that we cannot choose how or when we are going to die, we can and do choose how we will live, and how we can maximize our strengths. We can take care

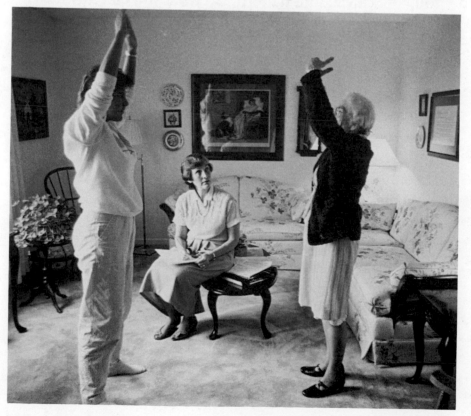

of these bodies of ours with active, positive decisions or abuse them and allow them to simply deteriorate by default.

Beth:

I used to think Grandma was immortal. As witty and agile as she was, I thought she'd never die. I told her once that if she ever thought she were going to die, she should call me up and I'd talk her out of it! She hasn't called me yet, thank goodness, but she *has* "called" me to lead a certain lifestyle.

I am forever grateful to Grandma for the model she has provided me. Thanks to her, my whole perception of growing older is different from the stereotypical view society holds. For me, the aging process is not something to be feared because I realize there are things to be done now to make my later years as fulfilling as possible.

My sincere hope is that you will be inspired by my grandmother, not discouraged. True, she has lived an extraordinary lifestyle which has kept her active, but it is never too late for any of us to make healthy changes in our lives. In co-authoring this book, I have definitely gained a renewed interest in my own health. I am reminded again how important it is to set the pattern now.

You, too, can set the pattern. Do what you can now to make life the best it can be. If, for some reason, you are *really* having doubts about setting a new pattern for your life, just call me up, and I'll talk you into it.

Grandma:

My concluding statement to you is made on what would have been my husband's and my 57th wedding anniversary. It is to emphasize again that you are at the right age to start something new, even if you are, as I am, approaching the finishing line.

Becoming more active by using some of the exercises we have suggested can indeed be of great consequence for you, not only the way you will feel physically, but how you will feel about yourself and accomplishing something new. To some it may seem that you are making very small steps. *You* know how great the steps are. "God is great in great things, but *very* great in small things."

"The art of living consists of dying young—as late in life as possible."—Anonymous

End Notes

Chapter 1—Three Is Not a Crowd

1. Lawrence E. Morehouse and Leonard Gross, *Total Fitness* (New York: Pocket Books, 1975), p. 21.

Chapter 2—Begin at the Beginning

2. Ted Kantner, interview, Hershey, Pennsylvania, summer 1985.

Chapter 5—Coordination and Balance

3. Lawrence J. Frankel and Betty Byrd Richard, *Be Alive as Long as You Live* (Charleston, West Virginia: Preventicare Publications, 1977), p. 230.

Chapter 7—Walking Your Own Mile

4. Gary D. Yanker, *Exercisewalking* (Chicago: Contemporary Books, Inc., 1983), p. 5.
5. *Ibid.,* p. 23.
6. Kenneth Cooper, *The Aerobics Way* (New York: Bantam Books, 1977), p. 192.

Facts: From the Office of Aging, U.S. Department of Health and Human Services.

—The degree of disability for seniors can be lessened through exercise.

—Exercise helps strengthen bone mass which is weakened in later age by osteoporosis.

—Exercise can increase muscular strength and endurance which deteriorates through inactivity.

—Exercise improves a person's joint flexibility and range of motion by keeping them loose and mobile.

—A sense of balance (potentially reducing chances of falling) is enhanced with exercise.

—Respiratory ability and efficiency (which may gradually decrease with age) can be improved with exercise.

—Arthritis cannot be eliminated but some of the painful symptoms can be relieved and flexibility increased.

—Improved circulation and a reduction in high blood pressure can be accomplished with exercise and diet.

—Mental status can be improved, and anxiety and the blues or mild depression can be relieved through exercise.

—The amount of oxygen (through improved circulation) can increase and enhance mental alertness.

Annotated Bibliography

Bailey, Covert. *Fit or Fat?* Boston: Houghton Mifflin Company, 1978.

The sub-title for this book reads, "A new way to health and fitness through nutrition and aerobic exercise." Bailey's approach to diets and, more specifically, to weight control, is that it is fat, not weight, that we should be concerned about. He insists that people get "overfat, not overweight," and that proper aerobic exercise can change muscles and alter the body's use of calories. A new and fascinating way to look at nutrition and exercise.

Baudhuin, John and Hawks, Linda. *Living Longer Living Better.* Minneapolis, Minnesota: Winston Press, Inc., 1983.

Emphasizing statistics that tell us that approximately 20 million Americans are 65 years and older, and how that will increase, this book looks at problems and challenges of the "surprises and unexpected gifts around the next corner" which can continue to make life worthwhile. Physical, spiritual, mental, social, and emotional components are a part of this "whole person" approach to aging. Dispels some common myths and fears about aging and gives practical advice for specific living skills.

Collingwood, Tom and Carkhuff, Robert R. *Get Fit For Living.* Amherst, Massachusetts: Human Resource Development Press, 1976.

This book tells how to assess your level of fitness, how to set goals for yourself in areas you want to improve and how to develop your own program of fitness. The authors use a continuing story of Jim and Sue to show how their program can work. Exercises are described and illustrated by drawings, and charts are shown which will help you to see your progress.

Cooper, Kenneth H. *The Aerobics Way.* New York: Bantam Books, 1977.

Dr. Cooper is hailed as the "man who started America running." A lot has been written proclaiming the benefits of preventive measures such as weight control, proper diet, eliminating the use of tobacco, etc., but this book is to update the guidelines that help you implement preventive medicine. There are age-adjusted, sex-adjusted, exercises, dietary recommendations and suggestions about weight control and even tips on how to quit smoking—all of which he says are necessary if you want to assure yourself of "maximal protection from one of the self-inflicted diseases in the Western hemisphere." (If you are interested in aerobics, his other books are excellent. *Aerobics, Aerobics for Women, The Aerobics Way,* and *The New Aerobics* can be found in most bookstores.)

Dychtwald, Ken. *Wellness and Health Promotion for the Elderly.* Rockville, Maryland: Aspen Publication, 1986.

An excellent resource for those working with older adults. Includes the work of many leading researchers, seminal thinkers, pioneering program designers, and key policy analysts. Emphasis is on offering information, resources, and programs for preventive health care and self-reliance.

Farquhar, John W. M.D. *The American Way of Life Need Not be Hazardous to Your Health.* New York: W. W. Norton and Company, 1978.

The title says it all! The author asks us not to assume that our lifestyle is a healthy one and makes a credible effort to demystify medicine and give us high quality health education. He talks about the usual concept of diet in more positive terms by calling it a healthy pattern of eating, and uses the idea of alternative food patterns. Methods of self-directed change that will help you live a healthier life and lower your risk of developing various diseases are carefully emphasized.

Frankel, Lawrence J. and Richard, Betty Byrd. *Be Alive as Long as You Live.* Charleston, West Virginia: Preventicare Publications, 1977.

This book is the result of a project called Preventicare, which addresses the goals and aspirations that can become a part of growing older with "reassuring poise, grace and equanimity." The sub-title, "Mobility Exercises for the Older Person," captures the goal of maximizing the strengths of older people.

Godfrey, Dr. Charles, and Feldman, Michael. *The Ageless Exercise Plan—A Complete Guide to Fitness After Fifty.* New York: McGraw-Hill Book Co., 1984.

A nicely written, attractive exercise guide for persons who would like to regain a healthy and active level of functioning or retain physical fitness. It emphasizes joint flexibility and safe, inexpensive ways of keeping fit for a lifetime. Designed for persons 50 and over, although a good guide for anyone who has not gotten into a regular exercise program.

Kuntzleman, Charles T. *The Complete Book of Walking.* New York: Pocket Books, 1979.

This author insists that walking is one of the best proven, enhancing and strengthening ways to change your life, and improve and keep your health. "It's the natural way to look and feel fantastic!" Full of illustrations, exercises for walkers, and even very specific walking tour maps of various cities.

Longacre, Doris Janzen. *More-with-Less Cookbook.* Scottdale, Pennsylvania: Herald Press, 1976.

This is not your ordinary cookbook. It evolved because the author along with many others felt that we as North Americans are over-fed and have an over-abundance of food in relation to the world's food needs. Recipes take up about two-thirds of the book. The remaining part has to do with learning to "enjoy more while eating less." "There is a way of wasting less, eating less, and spending less which gives us not less but more" . . . "More joy, more peace, less guilt; more physical stamina, less overweight and obesity; more to share and less to hoard for ourselves." You should not be without this book which is meant to be read carefully and thoughtfully. It is a great recipe book as well.

Morehouse, Laurence E., and Gross, Leonard. *Total Fitness.* New York: Pocket Books, 1975.

Regardless of your age, this little book promises you will feel fit and slow down the aging process in a minimum of time. Dispels numerous myths such as "protein makes you strong" and "sweating gets you in shape." The author writes in an easy reading style and makes you feel as though you really can improve your physical condition if you follow his advice. He has a simple formula for stopping what he calls "creeping obesity" by using 300 activity calories each day and eliminating 100 calories.

Morrissey, Barbara G. *Therapeutic Nutrition.* Philadelphia: J. B. Lippincott Company, 1984.

Although this is written with clinical nurses in mind, the author acknowledges the awareness of the general public regarding the role nutrition plays in promoting health. An assessment of nutritional status and what can be done to enhance recovery and promote health are part of this book. Dietary alterations to suit individual life-styles are included. These adjustments throughout the life cycle, including diets for the aging, are outlined.

Nelson, Eugene C., D.Sc., *et. al. Medical and Health Guide for People Over 50.* Glenview, Illinois: Scott, Foresman and Co., and Washington, D.C.: American Association of Retired Persons, 1986.

Official text for "Staying Healthy After 50," a nationwide health promotion program sponsored by AARP, the American Red Cross, and the Dartmouth Institute for Better Health. Tells how to use self-care techniques for treating chronic medical conditions, develop methods for handling stress, improve health through physical fitness (a few illustrated exercises included) and proper diet, become a more informed and cost-conscious health consumer, and maintain your own health and medical records.

Pollock, Wilmore and Fox III. *Health and Fitness Through Physical Activity.* New York: John Wiley and Sons, 1978.

For the serious student of health and fitness, this book tells how exercise programs are developed and how those are an integral part of preventive medicine. There are many research findings, exercise physiology, and fitness evaluation procedures included. Nutrition, special consideration for various levels of fitness and health, and specific rehabilitation programs are outlined. An excellent resource for persons concerned with exercise physiology and working with special needs.

Sheehan, Dr. George. *Dr. Sheehan on Fitness.* New York: Simon and Schuster, Inc, 1983.

This is not the author's first book and the emphasis is again on the belief that fitness has everything to do with the quantity and quality of life. This means a life full of activity, a fitness formula that can be made to fit you, as well as how to deal with stress. His chapter "On Aging" is especially well written. Although running is emphasized, the ideas regarding health and activity are very helpful and practical.

Yanker, Gary D. *Exercisewalking.* Chicago: Contemporary Books, Inc, 1983.

If there is any doubt in your mind that walking is not good for you, in fact one of the best exercises you can do, just read this book! You can convert the walking you already do to exercise routines of walking that will indeed keep you healthy. "Walkers are not fanatics like other sports enthusiasts . . . Walking itself calms you down and gives you an even-handed view of life and exercise."

Journals and Magazines

Modern Maturity—Published bi-monthly by the American Association of Retired Persons (AARP), 215 Long Beach Blvd., Long Beach, CA, 90801.

"Dedicated to helping all older men and women achieve independence, dignity and purpose." A truly worthwhile magazine!

Generations—Quarterly Journal of the American Society on Aging, 833 Market St., Room 516, San Francisco, CA, 94103.

An up-to-date journal on developments and issues related to aging. It promotes networking, reflects the national scope and impact that programs, policies, advocates and all levels of government have on aging and vice versa. This journal would be extremely helpful to those directly involved in the issues related to older persons.

Geriatric Nursing, The American Journal of Care for the Aging—Published bi-monthly by the American Journal of Nursing Company, 555 West 57th St., New York, NY 10019 (Subscription Department—Geriatric Nursing).

This journal is a must for anyone involved in direct nursing care of the aging. Although it is written primarily to a nursing audience, there are many articles appearing with each issue that will be helpful to anyone responsible for and interested in the aging.

About the Authors

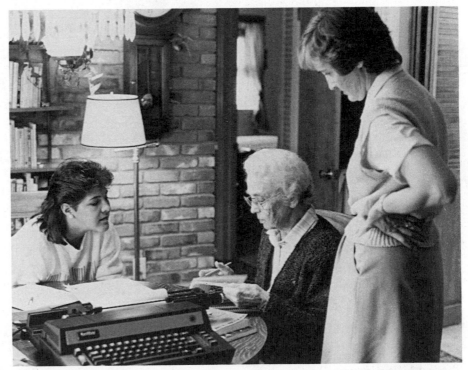

Naomi Lederach (right) is director of Education at Philhaven Hospital, a mental health facility near Mt. Gretna, Pennsylvania. For 12 years she was a nursing instructor at Hesston College in Hesston, Kansas. Naomi and her husband, John, regularly lead seminars on marriage and family life issues. They are the parents of three grown children, John Paul, Philip, and Beth. They also have three grandchildren.

Nona Kauffman (center) lives at Greencroft Center, Goshen, Indiana, where she assists in many activities, does occasional tutoring, speaks at banquets and programs, and teaches Sunday school. She and her late husband, Amsa, spent most of their adult lives in Goshen, where he pastored and she taught school. She also taught in Iowa and Texas. She is the mother of three daughters: Miriam Byler, Naomi Lederach, and Judy Kennel.

Beth Lederach (left) is a graduate student in education in Philadelphia, Pennsylvania. For three years she taught English and directed the dance-drill team, the Tigerettes, at Sam Houston Senior High in Houston, Texas. In 1986, she was chosen "Outstanding Young Educator" from among 10,000 teachers in the Houston school district.